A POISONED
MIND

A POISONED MIND

A POPULAR PATH TO UNDERSTANDING EPIGENETICS

*How Scientists and Sages can Clean your Genes,
and How to Do-It-Yourself*

BY

KURT GASSNER

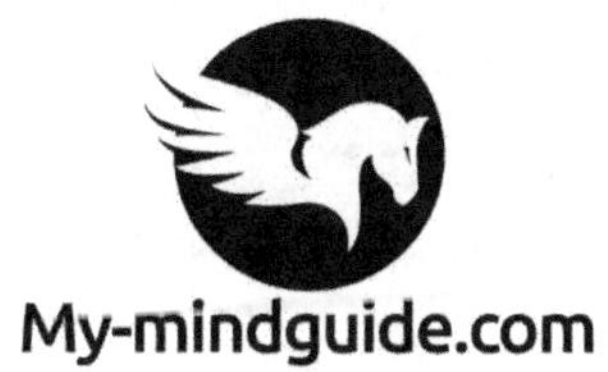

My-mindguide.com

A Poisoned Mind
Kurt Gassner

Impressum
My-mindguide – The publishing trademarke of trendguide Capital GmbH, Klenzestr. 42a, 80469 Munich, Germany.

Reg. Nr. HRB Munich 206639, VAT 152 123 159, CEO: Kurt Friedrich Gassner
Web: www.my-mindguide.com, mail: gassner@my-mindguide.com

Paperback ISBN: 978-3-98793-919-8
Hardback ISBN: 978-3-98793-995-2

Table of Contents

Foreword - My Reason Why

When you find something that changes your life,
what do you do?

For me, there's only one answer. Share it.

Share it in the most powerful, direct, and widespread way you can. Use all the means and methods at your disposal to get the message of hope and change out to those human beings that will benefit the most from it. You've learned it the hard way, and for a good reason. Make it easier for others.

This was what happened in my personal discovery of epigenetics. When I learned a little, connecting the dots became effortless. The more I learned, the more diverse aspects of my life, health, and spiritual practice started falling into place, setting up for a miracle that was to take place. Now, I keep learning. I sit back in awe and wonder about the sages and the scientists, and how we are learning more of life's great story.

I wrote this book to spread the transformative power that a thorough and holistic understanding of epigenetics can bring to people's lives. Our legacy is what we leave in others' heads and hearts, not the assets on our will, nor the cash in our bank.

All I hope is that this book leaves an imprint in your mind and imparts a spark to your heart. If it succeeds in doing so, then I know that you and your descendants will embark on a happier and healthier future.

How did learning of epigenetics change your life?

To understand this, and to fuel your full appreciation of this book, I first need to tell you a story. Don't worry—this is not my full life story. I won't bore you with an old man's tales, but bear with me, as this requires travelling all the back to the very beginning.

As with many people my age, I was born affected by the great tragedies and terrors of World War II. I was not involved in the war (I'm not that old!), nor did I ever witness conflict first-hand. However, I was born to a father whose whole life was influenced and directed by his experiences of the war-torn years. He was born in Ried, Austria in 1927, meaning he was of schooling age during the Nazi rise to power, and during its brief but tragic rule.

My father was a bright boy, with the outward appearance and genetics that Hitler happened to be after. As such, he was accepted into a National Political Institute of Education (German: *Nationalpolitische Erziehungsanstalten*; commonly abbreviated to 'Napola'). These were elite German boarding schools, partly modelled on the British boarding school; however, the curriculum was designed by the Schutzstaffel or 'SS', the paramilitary organisation that carried out much of the political, social, and military aims of the Nazi leadership. The schooling staff were of this population, as well. Nelson Mandela once said, "Education is the most powerful weapon which you can use to change the world." Unfortunately, the Nazis were also well aware of this fact and made the indoctrination of the German youth paramount to their plans for changing the world, Napola was the epicentre of this.

My father spent five years in a Napola school in Dresden, from the ages of 12 to 17, where he quickly grew into a young man. Over this time, he was comprehensively conditioned into the belief system and propaganda of the Nazi regime. This imprint never left him and remained embedded in his being even as he sat in approached his deathbed.

Like many Napola students, my father was also a child soldier. In the last few months of the war, a desperate Fuhrer called on the student reserves to fight to the last man (or boy) for the survival of the Third Reich. So, ill-equipped, under-trained, and underage, my father fought in the last Battle of Hungary (SS Totenkopf) and was injured in the process.

Through all this chaos, my father was still a family man. He met a woman, fell in love, and had children. It's true what they say… our fathers are our first teachers and our first heroes. We emulate them before we are even self-aware. As with most boys growing up, I admired my father, respected him, listened to his opinions, and sought to imitate him. I adopted his views on the racial superiority of Aryans, the hierarchy of races beneath that, and the great Jewish conspiracy to disrupt and overthrow European civilisation, not to mention a rather rosy view of what previous German generations had done to try and stop the Jews in their concerted effort. These views established the substrate of my beliefs and world-forming. It was simply the diet of thoughts that was offered to my young mind. I was conditioned by my parents (as we all are), and I have no shame in admitting that. However, I can also see how my life might have been easier and smoother had I been fed a different set of beliefs.

By all conventional standards, and through little fault of my own, I developed into a racist child with beliefs rooted in dark conspiracy theories. The stress and toxicity that oppression internalises into the psyche and body was also growing within me. A chain of negative thought patterns that would later turn into negative habits with the ability to damage our genes had already been planted in me.

Our fathers might be our superheroes for some time, but one of the most significant moments of self-development in child psychology is witnessing and understanding the failure or fallibility of our parents. This is essentially a death of the parental god, which causes us to see the world through an entirely new vantage point. When I turned 15, after spending more time in school exploring both history and science, I started questioning my father's viewpoints, and began challenging his beliefs. Then, at age 21, I started to travel—first throughout Europe, then worldwide. In the Bible, Paul had the scales of prejudice fall from his eyes whilst on the road, and so it was for me.

I spent time in Africa where I understood that genetics wasn't the culprit in holding African people back from prosperity or successes; it was due to structural, historical, and political reasons, many of which—but not all—resulted from the after-effects of European action and disruption on the continent.

I travelled throughout America and worked as creative director in New York at the age of 28. There, I stayed for several weeks with a Jewish family, which made it clear that Jewish people were every bit as loving, intelligent, generous, graceful, and well-intentioned as the rest of us, and in this particular family's case, quite a lot more. These trips and experiences represented the gradual erosion of the concrete conditioning that my father had bequeathed to me. They were essential to me shedding a racist and toxic legacy, and I feel richer for having walked that path out of darkness and into light.

Life carried on, and I built a career, founded and sold businesses, stumbled upon the love of my life, and started my own family. But amongst all this, upon witnessing certain scenes, my paternal prejudices somehow managed to sneak back into my mind. Of course, I didn't listen to these thoughts for more than a moment, and I quickly shot them down with multiple life examples and moral points. However, a tiny echo remained—a psycho-cultural hangover from my father that had not been fully resolved.

Could you ever truly heal? Could you ever move beyond your cultural and genetic inheritance?

Yes.

Covid-19 was a reckoning for all of us. For better or for worse, it provided an opportunity for a total break from old patterns—a chance to set a new course as an individual, as a family, as a country, and as a world. In the few years prior, I had been enjoying partial retirement by travelling extensively with my wife. I was searching for—and for the most part, finding—fulfilment in the great world out there, seeing many lands and meeting many people, squeezing each drop of experience out of the fruit of life. When Covid-19 came along, as with everyone else, my external explorations were forced to cease. What began after was much richer and more rewarding. My focus shifted from the external to the internal; my exploration continued within rather than without.

Pre-Covid-19, I had a meeting with someone who opened the door to epigenetics for me. I met Professor Johannes Huber, a leading physician and inspirational thinker in Austria, who has been referred to as the 'hormone pope' and is a leader in endocrinology and women's medicine. He is also an expert in the developing field of epigenetics. We engaged in lengthy conversations, during which I tried to absorb as much information as possible so I could later explore the concepts in my own research. During these conversations, I felt like my life was a jigsaw puzzle, steadily being solved as we discussed my past and his research.

He suggested a particular reading to me, which instantly transported me back to my childhood and into the feelings behind the toxic beliefs I adopted from my father. It was almost as if my heart and head physically clicked while the meaning of the words on the page slowly sank into my psyche. The research paper was from New York's Mount Sinai hospital[1], where the study had evidence suggesting that the genes of children of Holocaust victims had marks that increased the likelihood of stress and personality disorders. Now, there is no shortage of evidence for how racism and xenophobia can lead to oppression and the infliction of violence. It's also evident how these racist beliefs are intergenerational, as parents tend to pass on specific beliefs to their offspring. That being said, there was never a genetic angle to this problem. Yet here it was. The

---

1 https://pubmed.ncbi.nlm.nih.gov/26410355/

latest scientific research demonstrated how those toxic beliefs, through stress and trauma, could be genetically imprinted across generations to spew poison and pain down through the years. Whilst violence happens in one direction, everyone is damaged in the process—both the victim and the perpetrator. I did not have the trauma of the Holocaust on my epigenome, but I *did* have hateful ideas pressed into my psychology, which held the same potential to damage me those around me. Though my lessons in travelling and living had been enough to change my mind on these topics, they had not been enough to rid my being of them.

Professor Huber lit a fire in me, and the time that Covid-19 provided me to explore this topic was like oxygen, allowing it to burn brighter and brighter. My world widened even as the restrictions tightened. I embraced a whole load of different practices and ways of healing. I completed extensive but remote courses in yoga and meditation teacher training, enough to advance from a novice to a confident practitioner and explorer of these fields.[2] I even facilitated a silent retreat at home with my daughter as part of my teacher education, where days of silence felt like ten years of learning. As my practices and capabilities deepened, my healing accelerated. I was learning to still my mind, move within my body, and wipe my psychological slate clean.

My journey into hypnotherapy most directly confronted my childhood conditioning.[3] The hateful imprints could be

---

2 Institute for spiritual psychology Dipl. Psych. Eckehard Wunderle; and Samayana Meditation Center, Bali, verified Yoga Teacher Training

3 Gabriel Palacios, Berne Suisse, Master Hypnose Therapist/ Coach certified in US / Suisse, Germany

accessed in those slow brainwave sessions, and, in serenity, the layers that had built-up could be removed, examined, and discarded. I was reprogramming myself and my mindset with what I truly believed in as an individual, rather than what my father had been taught to believe before me. My meditation practice worked in concert with the hypnotherapy, where, in peace and stillness, my psyche could reintegrate into its new, more loving form. The terrible thoughts and the insidious instincts simply weren't there anymore. They had fallen away from my psyche, and likely off my epigenome. I felt cleansed and powerful in my newfound ability to act under my own agency, detached from my dad's destiny. I felt free.

The seed had been sown in my mind, but the real work came about during these modes of healing, and in changing my lifestyle. I had listened to the scientist, learned from the practices of the sages, and there I was, cleaning my genes.

The headline of this process was in erasing the intergenerational hate that had haunted me though life, but this was by no means the sole improvement that I experienced. I had more energy, physically and mentally; my focus and mood levels both increased, and persistent pains and problems that had set in as old age advanced began to retreat. When we were able to see other people again, they would often comment on my renewed vitality. Indeed, with my newfound perspective and practices, I was able to contribute to others' lives and help people overcome their obstacles, rather than being fixated on my own. It was clear to me that this was all because I had systematically and scientifically understood the roots of my problems—those layered on my epigenome in childhood—and had then acted using a combination of cutting-edge science and ancient wisdom to lift those ills in ways I'd never even contemplated before.

What was perhaps most rewarding during this whole process was sharing this healing journey with my daughter. We learned epigenetics and meditated together, compared notes, shared deep moments, and instituted positive life practices that I know will continue long after I'm gone. And this was my most direct legacy. My cultural, lifestyle, and epigenetic legacy to my children is totally different and far more enlightened than that which was left for me. This is how we evolve as humans. We leave our children in better places than we were left.

But what's the use in keeping this knowledge for the benefit of my own blood, if she and her own children grow up in a world where the latent power in epigenetics is not well-known or put to good use? What's the use if our grandchildren grow up in a world where environmental toxins are still present in our air, water, and food, where the full damage of mental stress is not recognised, and where our epigenome worsens with our climate? We need new perspectives on how to live, and new ways of rediscovering old knowledge. What wisdom we do find we must share, quickly and powerfully, for the benefit of all.

And so, we return to why I published this, back to where we started, and so onwards to the true beginning of this book.

Part One

The Science of Epigenetics

Epigenetics

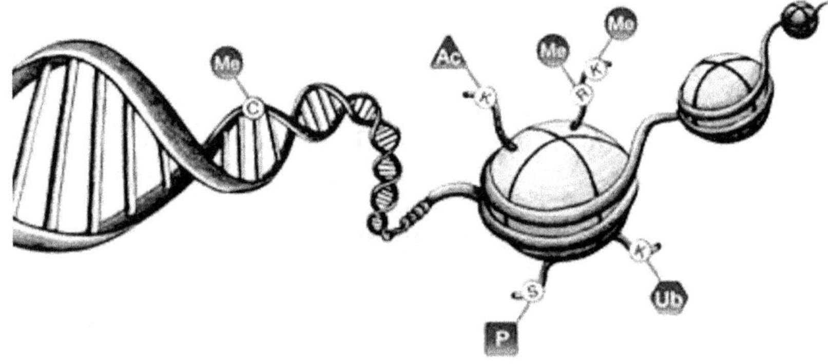

My-mindguide.com

Introduction - Genetics and Epigenetics - What's the difference and why does it matter?

What does the first book of the Bible have to do with genetics? Well, genesis and genetics clearly share a common root. As with most western scientific terms, we need to look back to ancient Greek. Genetics comes from γενετικός or *genetikos*, which means *genitive or generative*. This Greek word initially evolved from γένεσις or *genesis*, which meaning *origin*.

In the Bible book of origins, God had six days of 'highly efficient' work in which he created light, the world, its seas and mountains, and all of its creatures, including man. From Darwin to DNA, we have been extending those days into millions—if not billions—of years of geological formation and biological evolution. Through our study of genetics, we have more closely examined the last two symbolic days of Genesis 1, where God created all living things.

The discipline of science that we have most closely linked to God—and life itself—is that of genetics. It is the study of our origins, as individuals, as populations, as a species, and as carbon-based lifeforms.

Such profound links and relations between genetics, life, science, and spirituality can be made fairly easily, and they have been made quite often in recent times too, particularly accompanying the successful sequencing of the human genome, completed in April 2003. Consider Francis Collins' quotations on the matter, who led the Human Genome Project: "The God of the Bible is also the God of the genome. He can be worshipped in the cathedral or in the laboratory." Bill Clinton, the United States president during much of the research work said, "We are learning the language in which God created life."

You may now begin to understand how people saw the Human Genome Project as a monumental and fundamental leap in human understanding. We were learning the language of the Gods—the language of life itself. The implications of learning this language, and perhaps to start to speak or even code in it, were recognised by other luminary figures of our times. Regarding what humans might be able to achieve with this newfound knowledge, Bill Gates said, "Eventually we'll be able to sequence the human genome and replicate how nature did intelligence in a carbon-based system."

Many had equated genetics to God; both held a similar set of attributes—namely omnipotence, omniscience, omnipresence. Genes and DNA were everywhere in all forms of life; they were all-knowing in the sense that by reading them, we might know everything about a lifeform. They were omnipotent in that genes held total power over the future of that lifeform. Grand ideas indeed.

Although these were grand ideas, two problems emerge. Firstly, this book's central concept is not genetics. And secondly, whilst genes are omnipresent, DNA (or maybe RNA) is to be found in every organism living on earth. They aren't omniscient nor omnipotent as described above, as other factors are at play.

The good news is that this book focuses on the other factors that are at play—that is, the additional parts of the equation of life, beyond the genetics of it all. We focus on that which is beyond what your genes can really say about you and how you'll turn out, which is epigenetics.

It's time to return to words and etymology. We already understand that genetics comes from genesis, meaning origin. That Greek prefix '*epi - ἐπι*' means *beyond, above,* or *additional to*. So, the word *epigenetics* in its entirety can be translated as *that which is beyond the originating parts*, However, this book will reveal the true and deeper meaning of the word, as well as its impact on humanity.

In the two decades after sequencing the human genome, we've come to realise that those leftovers in the equation of life are rather more important than we'd first realised. Epigenetics, or the environmental factors that affect the expression of genes, has been credited by some scientists as accounting for nearly 50% of the equation of life's outcomes.

First, when something is likely responsible for up to 50% of the end result of a process, it's probably worth paying attention to.

Second, our gene sequences—our DNA—are fixed. They are predetermined by the sperm and the egg that met and fused to form our zygote, our primal cell. It's written code that—excepting possible future gene editing technology like CRISPR—cannot be changed whether we like it or not. But the same is not true of epigenetics. The environment that influences the expression of our genes is very much within our power to worsen or improve, all of which influences the course of our lives.

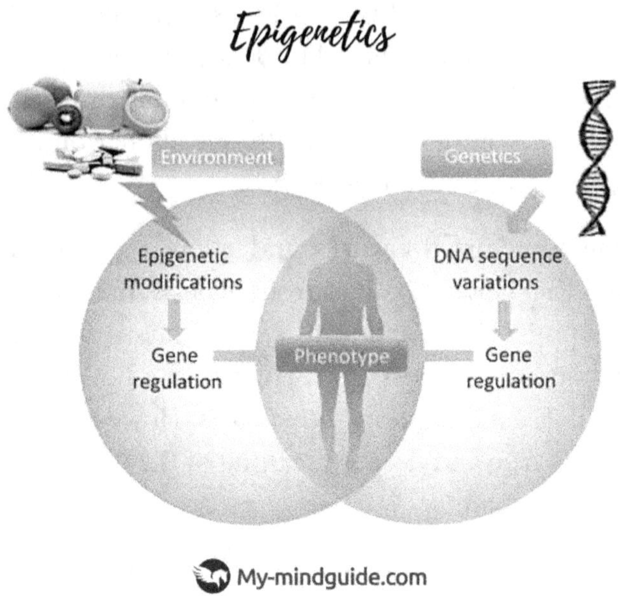

There are two vital points to gather and emphasise here.

That is why epigenetics is the focus of this book, as understanding it and putting its mechanics to good use ensures that, as Winston Churchill put it, "We are still masters of our fate. We are still captain of our souls."

Now, before we get too deep into the science and its development over the past century or so, a couple of explanatory metaphors may help clear the water. Metaphors in science are common, and the more complex or cutting-edge the science is, the greater the need for relatable ways of thinking about science. My favourite metaphors for the difference between genetics and epigenetics involve theatres and libraries.

Let's tackle drama first. Every play has a script—a fixed set of words that the actors will say in a fixed order. Let's take

Shakespeare's *Hamlet* as an example, focusing on one particular quotation concerning man and his place in the world:

"What a piece of work is a man, how noble in reason, how infinite in faculties, in form and moving How express and admirable; in action how like an angel, in apprehension how like a god: the beauty of the world, the paragon of animals—and yet, to me, what is this quintessence of dust?"

Hamlet will always say these words in Act 2, Scene 2. There are no deviations. Our genetics are the same. Across all the performances of our cells and across all its new versions in our body, these lines of code will be replicated. Interestingly, there may be a couple of times when the actor garbles the words, mistakes the line, or forgets. That's when mutations and potential problems, like cancerous growths, can occur.

However, when performing these lines, the actor may shout them in agony to the heavens, or he may whisper them to the ground in desperation. He may even look the audience in the eye and deliver them with a knowing wink. He could be dressed as a Scandinavian Prince in the late Middle Ages, a cowboy in the Wild-West, or even a spaceman. 'He' could even be a 'she' in an all-female production.

The theatre company makes these decisions, alongside the director, the cast, and the stage and costume designers. The same words will be said, but they can be said in a million different ways, all of which will leave the audience feeling a very different way when the curtain closes. Our epigenetics perform in this exact manner, where the script can be altered by conditional and environmental factors. It's crucial to note that we've all been given our script, but thankfully, its performance is very much up to us. For example, our parents make choices in raising us that determine when and where the play is set, how the lines are said, and how the audience (ultimately us) feels about the show.

Now, you can begin to understand why genetics alone is not enough. You can't comprehend Shakespeare based on the script alone; you have to learn from real performances, and perform it yourself, too, if you want to gain a deeper more thorough and authentic understanding of the play as a whole.

Drama doesn't happen on paper. As the great bard himself said, "The whole world is a stage." In the case of this metaphor and epigenetics, he was more correct than he could have ever realised.

Epigenetics

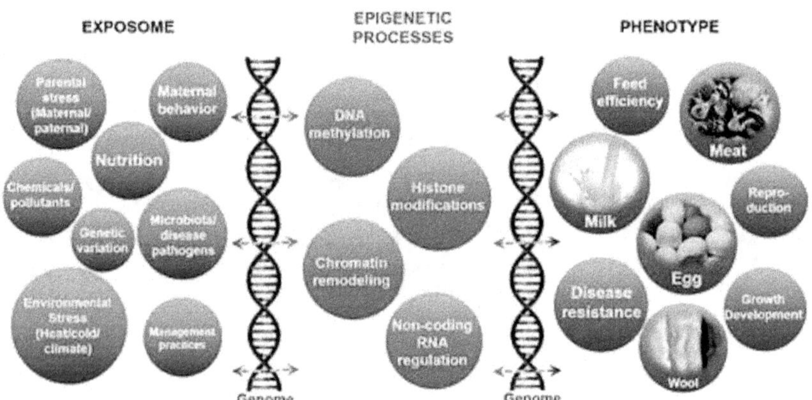

My-mindguide.com

1.1

A Whistlestop Tour of Genetics - what we've learned

Before we can come to understand epigenetics deeply, it is important to thoroughly explore genetics first. After all, to learn about *beyond-X*, we must know about *X* itself.

Note that this is merely a whistlestop tour, and by no means a full history of the discipline, as this is not the core focus of the book, and there are far more qualified people who can explain the development of the study in more depth than I can. This will give you an understanding of the journey humans have embarked on over the last two centuries in hopes of uncovering more information about genetics.

Imre Festetics, a Hungarian nobleman scientist, was the first to coin the word *genetics*. In 1819, he published *Die genetische Gesätze der Natur - The Genetic Law of Nature*. The four major laws he outlined in this book are as follows:

1. Healthy plants and robust animals are able to propagate and inherit their specific characteristics. → *Healthy organisms will bestow traits to their children and receive them from their parents.*

2. Traits of grandparents that differ from those of the immediate progeny may reappear in later generations. → *Traits may skip a generation, or 2.*

3. Animals possessing desirable traits that have been inherited over many generations can sometimes have offspring with divergent traits. Such progeny are variants of nature and are unsuitable for further propagation if the aim is the heredity of specific traits. → *Mutations can occur, kids will have some different traits than their parents*

4. A precondition for successful application of inbreeding is scrupulous selection of stock animals. → *'Good' genes can lead to 'good' traits.*

So, here is the entrance floor of the skyscraper (still under construction) of modern genetic knowledge. Next, we have Gregor Mendel, also known as the Father of Modern Genetics. Mendel was a polymath monk who lived in Moravia—today's Czech Republic. He was a meteorologist, mathematician, and, crucially for us, a biologist, too.

Mendel was a man of plants—pea plants to be specific. He bred, hybridised, and studied the different attributes of these plants from the vantage point of a mathematician, considering the importance of probability in outcome. He presented his core paper in 1866, *Verhandlungen des naturforschenden Vereines in Brünn,* or *Experiments on Plant Hybridization,* to the natural history society of Brno. Three discoveries, later termed *laws,* came out of his paper:

1. The Law of Segregation: Each inherited trait is defined by a gene pair. Parental genes are randomly separated to the sex

cells so that sex cells contain only one gene of the pair. Therefore, offspring inherit one genetic allele from each parent when sex cells unite in fertilisation. → *A child will receive half a set of genes from each parent, making a pair.*

2. The Law of Independent Assortment: Genes for different traits are sorted separately from one another so that the inheritance of one trait is not dependent on the inheritance of another. → *Receiving one allele ('half-gene') from a parent does not make receiving another 'half-gene' more or less likely.*

3. The Law of Dominance: An organism with alternate forms of a gene will express the form that is dominant. → *Some genes dominate the expression of others when in a pair.*

For what could be seen as one giant leap for all mankind in decoding the language of God, it received a couple local newspaper by-lines. To the world, at that time, it was merely a paper on the details of breeding plants and not much else.

For the next 35 years, Mendel continued to say his prayers and breed his plants until he died in 1884. If no one else understood the significance, he did: "My time will come," he reportedly told a friend.

There are two major theories for human discovery and invention. First, the *heroic theory*, where a great genius with brilliant insight and foresight single-handedly pushes forward the limits of human knowledge. Second, the *multiple discovery theory*, where a discovery or invention requires a comprehensive set of preconditions, previous discoveries, and ways of thinking, and when those are all present in a society, then multiple people will near simultaneously make that breakthrough. The beginning of genetics is a case study for both of these theories.

On the one hand, there is the lone hero, Gregor Mendel, who discovered the probabilistic mechanics underpinning the inheritance of evolutionary traits who stands (almost) alone in 1865 with his specific scientific research. But then we see a perfect example of the alternate hypothesis in the multiple (re) discovery of his work.

Over just two months in 1900, a Dutchman, Hugo de Vries, a German, Carl Correns, and an Austrian, Erich von Tschermak, all—to a greater or lesser degree—independently duplicated the research and writings of Gregor Mendel. When they came to read Mendel's previous work, they understood how he had got there first, and credited him with the discovery. The time for Mendel's brilliance was finally rip, and the study of genetics could take off at last.

A few years earlier, another under-appreciated breakthrough had been made. Swiss chemist, Johann Friedrich Miescher, had discovered a strange protein substance which separated out of cells when an acid was added. He labelled this substance *nuclein*, which is where the term *nucleic acid* comes from, as well as *nucleus*, where the DNA is stored in a cell. Over the next 40 years, scientists delved more and more closely into this *nuclein*, during which they discovered more about the nucleus' role in the reproduction of cells, and in how there is also genetic information (now known as RNA) in the cytoplasm (the rest of the cell).

In 1944, the *transforming principle*—today's DNA—was isolated from the nucleus as the primary genetic information in the Avery–MacLeod–McCarty experiment. So, in a hundred years or so, we had understood the birth of a cell, looked inside the cell and found the nucleus, and looked inside the nucleus and found DNA. Then, in 1953, another headline discovery rolled in when James Watson, Francis Crick, and Rosalind Franklin uncovered the structure of DNA in its double helix form.

Now, we head into the period of incremental and intensive scientific discovery. This is where different research teams around the world explored various aspects of genetics in multiple ways, all reporting their findings to each other through improved practises of scientific review and communication. The discoveries are incremental in that they steadily stand on the shoulders of other discoveries. They are less likely to be great leaps as with earlier pioneers and are better categorised as contributions. Still, there are always scientific events that make the headlines, and here they are, for some context:

In 1972, Walter Fiers and his team at Ghent University were the first to determine the sequence of a gene. In 1977, Fred Sanger, Walter Gilbert, and Allan Maxam sequences the entire genome of a bacterium. In 1982, we saw some of the first commercial applications of genetics; the FDA approved the release and use of the first genetically engineered human insulin, helping diabetics worldwide get the vital treatment they need. And with Type-2 diabetes soaring due to mass obesity in Western countries, this innovation couldn't have been better timed.

In 1985, Alec Jeffreys explained to the world the first method for DNA fingerprinting. In 1997, a sickly sheep named Dolly was born—the world's first mammalian clone. And as previously discussed, in 2003, the Human Genome Project was successfully completed with the full sequencing of our own DNA. This was a genuine landmark achievement, but only the start of understanding why we are the way we are.

The rolling juggernaut that is modern-day scientific research keeps rolling on, seemingly speeding up at an exponential rate. In 2021, scientists from Oxford University[4] developed a method to see—with far greater accuracy—how DNA forms large scale structures within a cell nucleus. This method allows for a magnification accuracy 1000 times greater than previously possible, providing the opportunity to measure contacts between different strands of DNA. As the press release stated, "If each letter of DNA was the size of a brick, each cell would contain roughly the number of bricks in a city (6 billion). Scientists are now able to work out which bricks are next to each other and see the fine details of how DNA forms structures inside cells, when previously they could only see the DNA 'architecture' on the scale of small buildings."

This discovery carries on the tradition that we've seen over the last couple of centuries in gazing ever more closely into the language of life. And with that, we make our way to the present day in humanity's quest to decode and speak the language of life.

---

4 https://www.ox.ac.uk/news/2021-06-09-scientists-make-dna-breakthrough-which-could-identify-why-some-people-are-more

Epigenetics

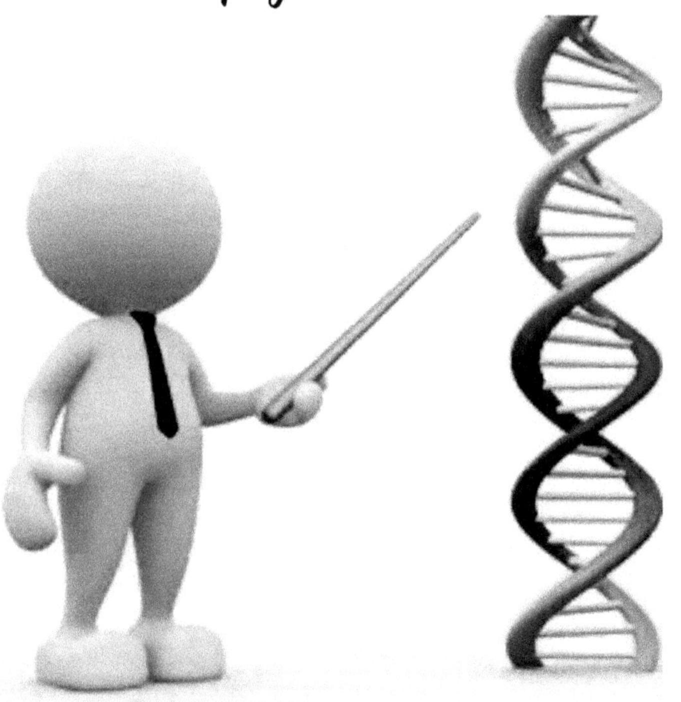

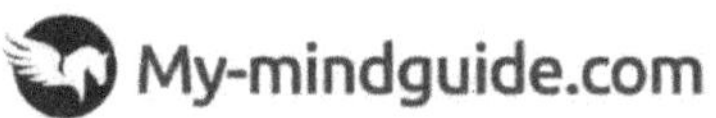

1.2

The Genetic Library - *Metaphors are a gene's best friend...*

Now you know a little about the developments in humanity's understanding of the coding language that we are all programmed in. But what about your own understanding? To get the most out of the rest of this book, you'll need a workable understanding of DNA—what it looks like, how it's structured, and the role it plays in the life of a cell. Note that this explanation is rather surface level, and certainly won't grant you a PhD in molecular biology. Still, it is important to gain a foundational comprehension of this concept before moving forward. And in that light, I'll call on the second metaphor that I'm comfortable with: libraries.

So, let's brace ourselves for a very extended analogy, and pretend that our body—our organism—is like the whole of human civilisation.

Then, let's consider each cell a human settlement—villages and towns. Each has its own industry or purpose. Some are mining towns, or farming villages responsible for producing useful resources. Others are manufacturing towns or service towns. Some settlements focus on decision-making, governing cities that help regulate the whole world, and even military barracks that will defend the civilisation against external threats. In all, there are about 200 different types of settlements, just as there are 200 types of cells in our body—each of varying size, and each serving its own unique purpose.

By the way, our civilisation is *huge*, with around 30 trills settlements—or cells—in total. Administering and maintaining such a large and complex organism is difficult and requires good systems to be developed over a long period. Thankfully, biological evolution over 3.5 billion years has provided us with systems capable of successfully governing large and complex organisms (or civilisations). But do remember that it all started with the local government of a single-celled organism—similar to the way in which a chief heads up a single village—before a complex civilisation could emerge.

That being said, these 30 trillion settlements are all common in one respect: they all have a state library. And since we are in this nation-free utopia, these settlements all have the same knowledge and information. That is, the books of each library in each settlement are all = identical and are arranged in the same order. This represents how each cell has a nucleus (the library), for storing genetic information or DNA (the books). We keep the same DNA (books) in every cell in our body. And when a new cell is created, the pages of each book are copied, and the new settlement is given its own library.

As always, there are a few exceptions to the rule. There are two known types of settlements that have no libraries. First, red blood cells have no nucleus. So, to extend the metaphor (perhaps further than it warrants), you might think of those cells as merchant caravans or trade galleys. They don't want or need to carry around all those books; they save space for more storage (haemoglobin), which allows for valuable goods (oxygen) to be carried around the world. The other type of cells with no nucleus library are known as keratinocytes, which are the outer, hardened cells of our skin, hair, and fingernails. This represents the outer wall, protecting our great civilisation from the dangerous outside world. And logically speaking, you wouldn't store precious books in your outer fortifications.

What is the purpose of this library? Well, the purpose of any library is to store knowledge. Each library acts as an archive for all civilisational knowledge. Its shelves contain the instruction manuals and laws detailing to the people how to act and behave, so that the whole civilisation can expand, flourish, and indeed start new civilisations (babies).

But back to the settlements and their libraries. Let's look at the architecture of the library and what's inside. The library is a big sphere, with a domed ceiling, and has two layers of walls—say for better insulation and protection from the elements. These are the inner and outer membranes of the nucleus. There are doors—or portals—into the library, which are the nuclear pores. Now, of course, these libraries don't use conventional books with spines and pages set against one another. They store information like the ancients: using a system of scrolls.

Before we can examine the scrolls, we must first look at how they are stored. The scrolls are stored on huge X-shaped shelves, where one shelf (i.e., a single *V*) links back-to-back with another *V*, thus forming an *X*. Interestingly, one *V*, and all its scrolls, come from the mother civilisation, whereas the other *V* comes from the father civilisation. In this way, the laws and information governing a civilisation are inherited from its parent civilisations. Scientists refer to our X-shelves as a pair of chromosomes. The average human (birth defects aside) has 23 *V*'s from their mother, and 23 *V*'s from their father.

So, on one of these V-shaped shelves, we have hundreds or thousands of treatises, but they are all stored on one long, single scroll. That scroll is wound around many reels to keep it orderly and in good condition. I find it easiest to picture the scroll as the paper receipts are printed on in supermarket tills, imagining that the roll of paper keeps extending onto multiple reels. The only other part to imagine is that the scroll also has twists in it, hence the double-helix shape of DNA. The 'paper' that the information is printed on is called the chromatin fibre.

So, in total, we have 46 long scrolls stored on 46 V-shaped shelves, which, in pairs, form an X. The scroll itself is our DNA, and if you rolled out each scroll until it were flat, its physical length would be about five centimetres, albeit only a few molecules wide. And so, all of our genetic information would be about two metres long when fully extended.

As mentioned, there are hundreds or thousands of treatises printed on each *V* shelf or chromosome, each treatise representing a single gene. The *V* shelf from the mother and the *V* shelf from the father contain a similar set of genes, but these genes are not identical. There are variations of the same scroll from the mother and the father. The scroll is in the same place, serves a similar function, and has a similar script on it, but it's not identical to the other. One of these variant scrolls is dominant, and the other recessive, meaning one scroll is focused on in the library, while the other gathers dust. The scientific term for the variant scrolls is *alleles*, and so, we have dominant alleles and recessive alleles.

To give some context and scale to our library collection, on average, a gene contains the instructions for three proteins to be made—or perhaps, three 'task manuals' for the people. The Human Genome Project estimates that there are about 20,000 genes in the nucleus of a human cell, or 20,000 treatises in our library, all stored on those 46 scrolls.

So, onto the language. What alphabet is used to write on these scrolls? Our alphabet has 26 letters; our computers use a binary system of 1's and 0's, but the language of life has four letters: A, C, G, and T—a quaternary system. And even then, these letters are always printed in the same pairs. A is printed on the same line as T, and G is printed on the same line as C. These are called base pairs, and a base pair represents a single line on our printed, twisted scroll. To give you an idea of scale, a base pair is composed of around 60 atoms. So, we are now at the smallest end of the biological scale. Any further and we are into atomic physics territory. Just as normal books vary in length, our genes vary, too. Some are structured like poems or short stories, with only a few thousand base pairs/lines, while others are structured like epic novels, requiring over two million lines to make their point.

All the people in these settlements have roles to perform, and they need to learn what to do and how to do it. And so, they rely on the information in the library to understand this. However, we don't want all the 'common people' in a settlement running in and out of our library, causing mischief and potentially damaging these precious records. These records need to be maintained as long as possible, as this will extend the lifetime of the civilisation or organism.

The double-walled membrane and the portals discussed earlier maintain access to the library. Only specific, learned citizens are allowed in the library—specialised 'academic' proteins. Indeed, our nucleus is not like a normal municipal lending library; it's a precious reference library. The scrolls can only be read on site; there is no lending allowed. Instead, there is a system of scribes, who, on request, look over the sacred scrolls, and transcribe the necessary information onto copied sheets. These cheaper copied sheets are then checked for errors, and after verification, are allowed out of the library and out into the rest of the cell to instruct the rest of the civilisation in its daily business. In this way, the contents of the library are protected, the common citizens get their instructions, and the civilisation can flourish into the distant future. In scientific language, these scribes are called *RNA polymerases*. They read the DNA and create mRNA versions of the genetic code that are sent out of the portals of the nucleus, and into the rest of the cell as instructions for the other proteins.

And so, we have the system of the Great Genetic Library. It's what got you here, and what keeps you here. Now, most of what we've discussed looks at this metaphor from a genetics perspective. We have a general, workable understanding of the system architecture of life, which is the design and basic functioning of an organism on Earth. And that's no mean feat.

However, we still haven't really mentioned epigenetics. You'll be glad to hear that the rest of this book is devoted to precisely that. However, don't forget this vital metaphor of libraries, for as you'll see, epigenetics also fits perfectly inside this civilisational analogy. We'll be getting back into the library, up onto its shelves, between its scrolls, and marking that same genetic paper, time and time again.

We've built up a foundational genetic understanding; now we can start the epigenetic dance on top of that floor of knowledge.

Epigenetics

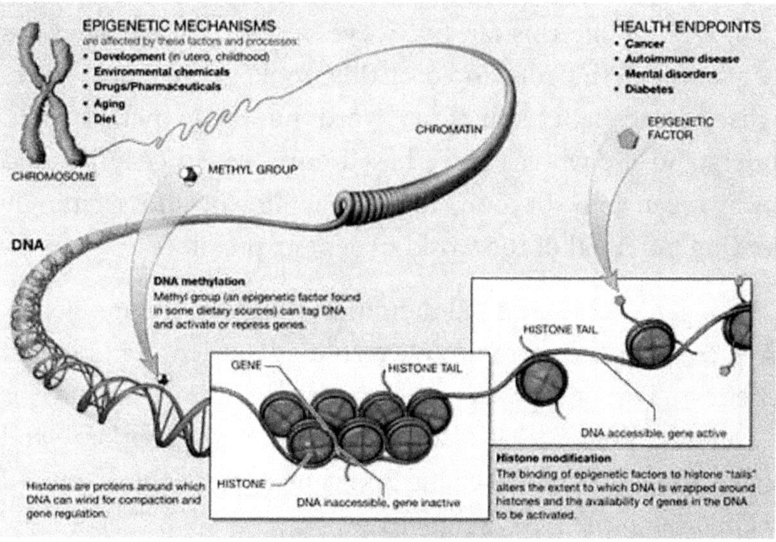

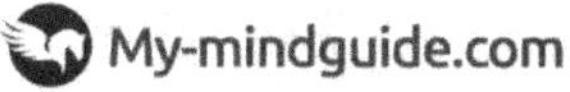

1.3

Getting 'epi'(c)

So, we've come this far, but we've only had a few sideways glances at the core topic of this book: epigenetics. We've focused on the latter half of that word thus far so that we could understand the whole. We've based ourselves in genetics, and now we can look beyond, into the emergent and seemingly dazzling potential of the world of gene-expression.

Let's get a more detailed definition of this evolving science, more so than the etymology we studied earlier, (i.e., beyond genetics). For our purposes, the best definition we have is as follows: Epigenetics is the study of both temporal and permanent (inheritable) changes in gene expression not caused by changes in the DNA sequence.

So, we are looking at biological processes that change how the cell reads and acts upon the instructions contained in the DNA sequence. Since they can be temporal or permanent, these changes may only last the lifetime of that cell, they may be passed on from one cell to its daughter cells, or these non-sequence changes may even be passed from one individual organism to its progeny. To jump back into our civilisation analogy, we are studying the systems of the library scribes, which serve to change the citizens' behaviour and may affect future offspring settlements and their own libraries, too.

If you prefer the stage metaphor, let's consider this: How can the director of the play influence the ways in which the actors say their lines, dress, or choose their props? What are the director's means of communicating these differences in artistic expression to their cast?

If all the cells in our bodies (excepting the two types mentioned earlier), have a full copy of all of our DNA—all the settlements have a library with the same instructions—then how do we end up with around 200 types of cells, rather than just a 30 trillion blob of the same cell type? The answer lies in epigenetics. By understanding the fundamental ways in which cells differentiate into varieties, we can open the door into how cells can express themselves in different ways. And that will answer our question above of how the director communicates with the actors in how to say their lines and what to dress up in.

Epigenetics

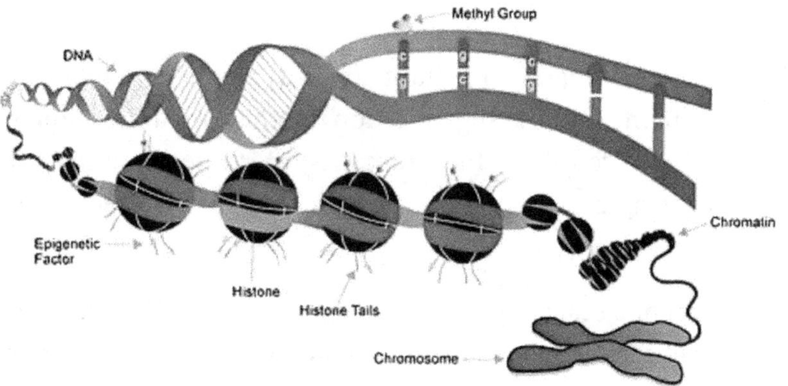

My-mindguide.com

1.4

——

The Great Variation Hunt - Epigenetics: Tinkering or Total Change

Now, we embark on a hunt for difference. Following on from the concluding question in the previous chapter, how do we account for the dramatic differences between the cells in a single organism, all of which share the exact same DNA?

And on one scale larger, how do we account for the dramatic differences in the behaviours and outcomes of individuals of a species or group, all of which share extremely similar DNA? (We share 99.9% of our DNA with all other humans.)

Well, thankfully, the hunt for the answers to these questions will take us directly and deeply into the realm of epigenetics.

Compared to our tour of breakthroughs in genetics, the tale of human advances in epigenetics is either quite a bit shorter and more substantially modern, or vastly more ancient, stemming to the very earliest shamans and witch doctors, clouded in the near impenetrable fog of human prehistory. This, of course, all depends on perspective and definition.

As we'll establish in the second section of this book, wisdom-keepers from every age have exhibited and extolled practices, diets, and detailed comprehensive systems for living that—as we understand today—would aid the healthy expression of our genes. The ancients understood the importance and impact of epigenetics, without actually understanding the precise molecular mechanics behind it—something we are still very much figuring out today. However, through meticulous observation and ancestral knowledge sharing, they *did* develop their own spiritual sketches for the epigenetic mechanism, both for an individual and between generations. But more on that later.

For the sake of this chapter, we'll consider the first—stricter—scientific perspective of epigenetics. So, rather than starting in the mists of time, we can begin in 1942, at Cambridge University, with a British developmental biologist by the name of Conrad Waddington.

Waddington was a developmental biologist who studied the way in which an embryo develops into a complex organism. Epigenesis—subtly different from epigenetics—was an earlier theory of development, which correctly asserted that organisms develop from generic cell types. The incorrect rival theory was known as *pre-formationism*, which stated that embryos were just miniature versions of mature organisms, and growth was all that was required. Waddington coined the term *epigenetics,* in partial reference to epigenesis, but also in how it concerned that which was beyond genetics.

Waddington was a fruit-fly fanatic. He performed the majority of his major experiments with drosophila, a species of fruit fly. He repeatedly heated generations of pupae, or fly eggs, to create a difference in the veins of their wings. Eventually, he successfully achieved this veinless trait in the population, without him having to provide that particular heat treatment to the developing flies. For him, this demonstrated how inheritable physical traits could be caused by repeated exposure to environmental factors. In sum, it was possible for the environment to change the expression of genes, passing these changes down throughout the generations.

Waddington was writing in the long shadow cast by two of the 19th century's most famous biologists. The first and foremost being Charles Darwin, and the second being Jean-Baptiste Lamarck. As we well know, Darwin's major contribution was the theory of natural selection—that random genetic mutations could affect an organism's ability to survive and procreate, and that survival of the fittest meant that the organisms with the most helpful mutations would more often succeed in life and reproduction. And so, a species evolves. Lamarck's big idea was the inheritance of acquired characteristics. This, in essence, was that in life, an organism would respond to its environment with a set of behaviour, which would cause physical traits to grow in use, or to wither in disuse. Then, when it came to kids, these changes would be reproduced in the organism's offspring. We likely have a solid understanding of Darwin's theory, but Lamarck's may need an example, and his most famous one was the giraffe. The precursor to the giraffe was born with a more normal length neck, but since it spent its life reaching up into high branches, its neck muscles extended, lengthening the vertebrae. When the pre-giraffe had kids, they came out with longer necks, inherited from their mother. And lo and behold, we have the modern giraffe.

Now, Lamarck's theory of acquired characteristics may sound more like one of Rudyard's Kipling's *Just So* animal stories, and that his giraffe example is right up there with "How the Camel Got His Hump" and "How the Leopard Got His Spots". Indeed, the vast majority of biologists came to see that Darwin was the father of their science, and Lamarck—well, perhaps more akin to a crazy uncle, which explains why you may not have heard of him until now.

Lamarck and Darwin represent two opposite ends of the spectrum in developmental theories, one stating that pure genetic mutation is what changes the heritable genome, whereas the other gives credit to behaviour and active training. Waddington's experiments and theories, along with the rest of modern genetics and epigenetics, sit somewhere between these two extremes. They are certainly more indebted to Darwin, but perhaps increasingly accepting of some of what Lamarck had to offer.

Waddington demonstrated that physical characteristics could be acquired and then eventually passed on, and the mechanism for this was epigenets—his own term. Waddington's verbal prowess was not just limited to coining terms though. This wonderful quotation explained his aims in scientific research: *"To explain the complex by the simple and discover more about the simple by studying the complex."* This is clearly our kind of scientist.

His greatest contribution in "explaining the complex by the simple" is his metaphor of the epigenetic landscape. This is how he saw the development of cells from generic embryo cells, down to all the highly specialised types of a cell that make-up a complex organism. He pictured a solid ball, starting at the top of a great hill. Beneath the ball, there is a system of hills and valleys. These hills may start as gentle rises and build into small ridges, but they will eventually grow into the sides of a great canyon. Now, the ball starts rolling down the hill. The formation of the slopes will determine where that ball rolls down. At the beginning, there will be some natural variation between where the ball rolls. But once the ball gets far down between a set of ridges, and then into the canyon, it becomes certain where that ball will end up.

Waddington saw our cells as balls. They start at a neutral point—the top of the hill—with the genetic potential to become any of our cells, as all our cells contain all our DNA. The ball starts rolling, and so, the cell starts developing and specialising. As the ball falls, its path and destination become more certain and more fixed—that is, the cell becomes more specialised. At the beginning of the journey, the cell can become many things, but as we progress down the slope, its options narrow, outfitting the cell for a given role. Our genes uphold the slopes of the landscape, and Waddington discovered that environmental factors can give that ball a push and change its developmental path. And he did this experimentally, by applying heat to those poor fruit fly pupae. For his early experimental demonstration of epigenetic changes, and his still-used theory of the epigenetic landscape, Waddington has come to be perceived as the father of epigenetics, in a smaller but similar way to the way in which we see Darwin as the father of evolutionary biology.

If there was a firstborn son of epigenetics, it might well be John Gurdon, another British developmental biologist, but this time, based in Oxford. And we can replace the flies with frogs—African clawed toads, to be precise. In essence, Gurdon was looking to see whether it was possible to push the ball up the landscape, and whether he could reach the starting hilltop again. Most of the research at the time said this wasn't possible, but, like Sisyphus with his boulder, he had an attempt regardless—many attempts, in fact.

Gurdon took cells from the intestine of adult frogs, and he removed their nucleus. He then took an unfertilised egg cell, which only had the female 'half' of the DNA, and removed its nucleus. He then put the intestine nucleus into the egg cell. So, he was essentially putting adult, developed, genetic information into the structure that is the first cell animals come from. It was like taking a ball from one of the deep canyons of an organism and placing it back onto another hilltop. Would it still be able to roll down?

After several attempts to refine the transplant technique, he was able to get that ball up onto that peak of life. And eventually, that first ball split into many more balls, which all rolled down the epigenetic landscape; they ended up mostly in the right places, and lo and behold, out came a living, breathing, ribbiting frog. The world's first adult-cloned animal in 1958.

This was an unbelievable breakthrough, and indeed, many didn't believe it at first. But by the time Dolly the Sheep was born from the same technique almost 40 years later, the doubters were long gone.

So, we can now see that a key part of a ball (the cell's nucleus) can be picked up and placed onto the landscape's peak. But what about the other possible journeys of a cell—all the different routes that can be taken down the same landscape (i.e., with the same DNA)? Is it possible to explore the ridges, the hills, and the valleys of a given DNA landscape?

The next giant leap of the proverbial frog did not come from a British scientist, but rather a Japanese one by the name of Shinya Yamanaka in 2006. Yamanaka was a physician by training, who was drawn into research. Rather than transplanting DNA into early egg cells, or lifting balls to other peaks, he wanted to explore the potential and possibility within Waddington's epigenetic landscape. You see, Yamanaka understood the difficult it took for a ball in a deep gorge at the end of its journey to be lifted across into the next gorge. However, if the ball was rolled further up the hill to where the cell's journey has not yet been clearly defined, it may be possible to roll it over a gentle rise—with enough of a push—and then let the ball roll down a different channel. In library terms, he wanted to turn a mining settlement into an agriculture settlement, or vice versa. In grand terms, he wanted to change the destiny of a cell.

Yamanaka identified 24 protein molecules present in stem cells, all of which are at the peak of the epigenetic landscape. These protein molecules are transcription factors (TFs). In the library, they are things that affect which scrolls are transcribed into copies to send out to the settlement. You might think of them as big labels on shelves, screaming, "Pick me! Pick me!" When these stem cell TFs are present, all the scribes pick the scrolls that are relevant to stem cells and send out those instructions from the library and out into the settlement.

Through rigorous testing, Yamanka isolated four key TFs— the four most eye-catching labels attached to the most crucial scrolls—that were sufficient to push a developed specialised adult cell back into a stem cell. Through inserting these epigenetic transcription factors known as OKSM, Yamanaka was able to roll the ball back to the top of the hill, changing the very destiny of a cell.

Like with John Gurdon, the sheer size of this breakthrough made it hard to believe for the scientific community at first. Yamanaka was dismissed by the world's top genetic labs as likely having made a mistake, or having misinterpreted the results. It was only when Rudolf Jaenisch, a renowned geneticist at MIT, announced that he had repeated the experiment and verified the results that this giant step was recognised. And within just five years, iPSCs—Yamanaka's term for these artificial stem cells—had become a common term known to anyone studying high-school biology. It's certainly a big deal when advanced scientific discoveries echo into the school classroom in that timeframe.

And in Waddington, Gurdon, and Yamanaka, we have traced a significant lineage in human understanding of the mechanisms of life. Waddington theorised how genetics— or their common DNA—did not decide the destiny of a cell, epigenetics did. Gurdon found it was possible to take a script from one cell and start the ball rolling in another, whilst Yamanaka discovered a path back up to explore Waddington's landscape of cellular life. It was appropriate that this journey of exploration was acknowledged in 2012 with a Nobel Prize, the two recipients: Gurdon and Yamanaka.

What does this journey mean for us? Well, it gives us a contextual understanding of major research advances in epigenetics. But far more importantly than this, it shows the sheer significance of epigenetics. Epigenetic factors are able to change the very nature of a cell. Two otherwise identical stomach lining cells have the same DNA and are specialised in the same way. With significant enough epigenetic inputs, or Yamanaka's four factors, we can turn one of the cells into a cell found in the heart, the liver, or the brain.

From a theatrical perspective, we can say that the same theatre company can stage two completely different performances, all whilst using the same script. Now, we can see how in epigenetics, we are not just limited to tinkering with the way one line is delivered, or similar minor alterations. Rather, in epigenetics, we have the potential to change life itself.

The effect is not just limited to the cellular level. Epigenetics has the potential to change the behaviour and lives of whole organisms. Perhaps the most colourful case study of this is in the collaboration between epigeneticists Danny Reinberg and Shelley L Berger, and the entomologist (ant fanatic) Jürgen Liebig. Liebig studied carpenter ants, a species with complex social structures and hierarchies. There are bullet-sized queens, who can reproduce and fly; majors, bean-sized, who defend the colony; and minors, grain-sized, who are foraging peasants that supply the colony's food. Reinberg and Berger injected an epigenetic-affecting chemical into the brains of developing major ants. The big surprise: these majors started to explore beyond the colony's walls and started foraging for food; they acted like minor ants. Their identity, function, and behaviour were altered purely through an epigenetic change in development. From this result, we can gather how epigenetics can change cells, cell alteration can change organisms, and changes to organisms can affect physical outcomes at our scale of life. Epigenetics is a force of change that can echo from the molecular up to the material. It's the engines of epigenetics that drive the wonderful variation that we see under the microscope in our own cells, and between organisms of the same species, which we observe with our own eyes, each and every day, in ant colonies and in human ones. So, if we want to change our role, to evolve our identity like the carpenter ants, then we must come to understand those engines of epigenetics.

Epigenetics

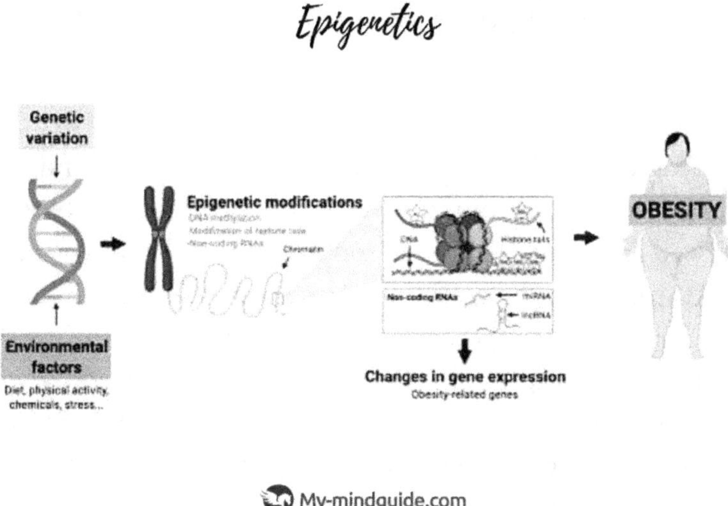

1.5

___

The Engines of Epigenetics

We've traced one line of epigenetic discovery and have learnt of the massive potential power of epigenetics, but we'd be remiss to point out some of the other major breakthroughs in the discipline. Not because we need a history lesson, but because these are the key known mechanisms that influence gene expression. Before we can be amazed by what epigenetics can achieve and how we might put it to good use, let's first understand how it works. We can build skyscrapers, but only on grounded knowledge.

So, in the next section of this book, we will discuss the potential external stimuli that can lead to these changes in gene expression—that is, how your external and internal environment affects your cells' behaviour. In other worse, let's discuss how your circumstances and choices affect your life—from a biological standpoint, of course. In this chapter, we will focus on what actually happens inside the library and on its shelves. What are the known mechanisms for altering DNA expression, and when and how did we discover them?

The two major epigenetic factors that we know of involve things called methyls and histones. Now, don't let the scientific terminology scare you. We won't venture too far out from the library metaphor we've already established.

We can start with DNA methylation, which was first discovered in Waddington's time in 1948. Rollin Hotchkiss, an American scientist working at the Rockefeller Institute, discovered the presence of methyls by examining DNA using paper chromatography. Methyls are small molecules of carbon and hydrogen. They are missing one hydrogen, which allows them to bind onto DNA molecules. For decades, scientists debated the purpose of these methyls in regard to DNA. In 1975, work by Riggs, Holliday, and Pugh on bacteria found evidence that the presence of methyls in DNA affected the expression of genes. They—and consequent researchers—found that the presence of methyl groups on genes repressed, or turned down, the expression of the genes.

Now, let's return to our library analogy. So, let's imagine we're looking out at those specific library scribes, who are walking up and down the shelves, selecting given precious scrolls, copying them onto expendable paper, and sending them out of the library as instructions for our settlement. We look at these dutiful and methodical servants of the settlement, and wonder: How do these scribes know which scrolls to pick?

Well, one of the ways is stapled ribbons. Some scrolls have red ribbons attached to parts of their length. They are stapled onto the paper in a pretty permanent way. Now, if we watch the scene more closely, we can see that the scribes seem to avoid the shelves and scrolls that have multiple red ribbons protruding from them. It might simply be because the scrolls are harder to access and transcribe with all those ribbons. Regardless, scrolls with red ribbons are selected less often, and so, fewer of their copies are sent out into the settlement.

At this point, another library official bustles past you, attaching and stapling the red ribbons to the scroll. His security lanyard has four letters and one number on it: DMNT-1.

These DMNT library officials are called DNA Methyltransferases. They are proteins in the nucleus responsible for methylating and demethylating DNA. Their existence, role, and impact were first studied in depth by scientists in the 1990s. There are three families or groupings of DMNT: Dnmt1, Dnmt3a, and Dnmt3b.

The Dnmt1 officials—let's refer to them as officials No.1— are responsible for maintenance. When the cell creates a new daughter cell with its own set of genetic instructions, these No.1 officials are responsible for ensuring that both the new and the old DNA have the same methylation patterns as the original DNA had before the new cell's generation. In the library, these officials are responsible for ensuring that the red ribbons are placed on the new scroll in the same positions as the previous one.

The impact of this is vital for us to understand. Ribbon patterns or methylation are inheritable from one cell to another, just like the base letters on the page. Therefore, things that affect methylation in cells can impact the organism across its whole lifetime, as those patterns are faithfully transcribed by one set of officials to another. What is more, there is mounting evidence that methylation can also be inherited across organisms, rather than just between cells of a single organism. In essence, not only do you inherit your parents' DNA (the writing on the scroll), but you are also likely to inherit at least parts of their methylation patterns (where the ribbons are placed).

If DMNT-1 is responsible for maintaining the same ribbon patterns, then who do we look to for changing these ribbon patterns? Well, no further than officials No.3-a and No.3-b. As we scan down the library shelves, we can see a few 3-a's walking around, pausing for consideration, and attaching their red ribbons in new places. But despite searching in most libraries across settlements, you'll struggle to find many 3-b's.

That's because Dnmt3a is the official in charge for the majority of the organism's lifetime. And as an adult reading this book, you'll only have significant amounts of Dnmt3b in your bone marrow, thyroid, and testes cells (if you have them). The role of 3b officials is most significant in the organism's early development. After that, they become fewer and far between. 3b's also have a specialist partner in the developing brain called Dnmt3L, but that's a little too in depth for the nature of our discussion.

Back in the library, we follow the work of one Dnmt3a. We watch her for a while to try and identify a pattern in the scrolls she selects for ribbon stapling. A few things emerge from our observation. First, there are whole lengths of scroll that she seems to almost totally avoid, nodding at them respectfully when she passes, and lowering her staple gun. Second, there are post-it notes that flutter around the library. When our 3a official passes one of the post-it notes that's attached to a scroll, she usually—but not always—staples a ribbon to it. Why is this the case?

Well, the areas that Dnmt3b tend to avoid methylating are known as CpG islands. CpG islands have a higher recurrence of the CpG gene pattern—a specific sequence of acid bases, or a recurring sentence on the scrolls. The locations and lengths of these CpG islands are very-well shared between mice and human DNA, which, alongside other evidence, suggests they are very important for proper development and maintenance of life. In essence, DMNTs know not to play around with these areas too heavily so as not to alter key sequences for healthy development in all mammals.

Now, what are those fluttering post-it notes? Those are *histone modifications*, also known as *histone marks*. But hold on a second. What's a histone, anyway? We can't get a working understanding of all this by hiding behind scientific terms. In our library, the histones are the little spools that the scrolls are wrapped around to keep the library's paper in reasonable order, and to prevent it from becoming a great spaghetti mess. Remember, if you stretched the human DNA contained in a single cell, it would come to approximately two metres in length. Since the average diameter of a nucleus in mammalian cells is six micrometres, and we could assume that the average length of a municipal library is 60 metres, then two metres of DNA would be equivalent to 120,000 kilometres of paper scrolls—or enough to wrap around the Earth three times. Now, we can understand why a good compact storage devices like histones are necessary.

Before we move onto histone modifications, let's dive a little deeper into the concept of the post-it notes that flutter around the library so we can truly appreciate the epigenetic power of histones themselves. When the paper is tightly wound around many scrolls, compacted closely together, the copier scribes find it hard to access these parts of the code, and so, they are transcribed less often, meaning their copies have a smaller impact on the activity of the cell. They are kind of like the dusty books on the top shelf that rarely get read. When certain genes are tightly packed around histones, their instructions and effects are less expressed by the cell and organism.

David Allis was one of the first people to think about histones in this way, and he was bucking conventional scientific wisdom at this point. Allis stated, *"Histones had been known as part of the inner scaffold for DNA for decades, but most biologists thought of these proteins merely as packaging, or stuffing, for genes."* This is a bit like scientists playing pass-the-parcel where they just rip open the outer wrapping to get at the big gift inside. The scientists are missing several tricks here, as most aspects of the game and meaningful prizes are contained in that very packaging in the structural layers. Allis saw the game for what it was. He wasn't a stranger to a poetic metaphor either: *"A skein of silk tangled into a ball has very different properties from that same skein extended; might the coiling or uncoiling of DNA change the activity of genes?"*

In 1966, Allis and his research team made a great discovery and a grant stride to answering his question. They found a protein that had the power to force open the DNA coil, or to unroll and then repackage the scrolls around spools. In his research, the genes that had been repackaged also expressed themselves differently. The scroll kept the same letters on it, but the instructions sent out to the cells had changed. He'd found and proven another epigenetic mechanism.

Allis was also involved with our post-it notes, or histone modifications. These fluttering notes attach themselves onto the spool of the scroll, acting like marker tags for our DNMTs and other similar officials. The main types of post-it notes are acetylation, methylation, and phosphorylation. So, the histones themselves can be marked by methyls. Acetyls are Allis' opening protein, meaning they neutralise the positive charge of the histone, thus reducing the tightness of the binding between the histone and DNA. This ultimately allows scribes to open the scrolls, ensuring they are read more frequently. Now, if DNA methylation turns down the impact of a gene, then the acetylation of histones turns up the volume of a gene. Allis also discovered that histone modifications are passed from a parent cell to a daughter cell when the cells divide. The post-it notes and their effects are therefore transferred into the new records when they are copied. They are less permanent than DNA methylation, which are stapled, but can still survive across cell reproduction.

We can refer to Allis and his colleagues as code breakers. They tried to crack our epigenetic code. The sequences of ribbons and post-it notes act as a type of cellular communication—a notation system on a molecular level. As previously discussed, sequencing the human genome was the first major step in coming to understand our genetic code. The scientists mentioned in this chapter attempted the same thing, but in epigenetics. The trouble is that, in genetics, we have a neat and stable script of four letters arranged in pairs. Sure, it's tricky to discern how that script comes to impact the whole organism, but we have one set of variables to account for. In epigenetics, on the other hand, we have several types of dynamics that can all influence the expression of DNA, and can all change over the lifetime of a single cell or organism.

We have many histone modifications, methylation patterns, and—a third, even less understood actor—non-coding RNA.

These epigenetic mechanisms relate and respond to each other in highly complex ways. It's not a case of histone modifications simply causing methylation, or vice versa; these elements have more complex multidirectional relationships with one another. It's a molecular-sized, ever-moving, and probabilistic puzzle.

This means that—just like you—our research scientists are standing in the library, trying to better understand how the post-it notes relate to ribbon stapling. Which one impacts the other; which patterns can emerge, and how permanent and inheritable are they? This is not yet a fixed science, widely agreed and immutably taught in the classroom. We are now on the cutting edge of current understanding where scientific debates and conflicting theories are rife.

We have just one more aspect of molecular-level epigenetics to cover, and for our purposes, it's perhaps the most important: inheritability. Our science story here involves a group of inbred yellow mice and a pioneering Australian researcher, Emma Whitelaw.

The yellow mice in question are called agouti mice. They have been inbred across hundreds of generations to have no variation in their DNA. The whole population, across all laboratories of the world, are genetically identical twins. And unsurprisingly, this inbred species comes with its own set of problems. They are prone to obesity, diabetes, cancer, and have abnormal yellow fur. These problems make them a great experimenting model for studying chronic diseases that afflict our industrialised society.

The yellow fur traits were driven by the dominant allele, *A*, whilst, normal fur is enabled by the recessive allele, *a*. What is strange is that genetically identical mice raised in the exact same laboratory conditions could have different shades of fur, from yellow, to mottled, to the normal black. How can that be when the *A* is dominant and should always be expressed? Whitelaw discovered that when the *A* gene becomes heavily methylated, the agouti gene is switched off, and the mice become a standard brown.

She and other fellow scientists then experimented using variables that would affect the methylation of this gene. These variables included diet, exposure to harmful chemicals, and ionising radiation. Changes in exposure to these variables impacted the methylation, thus impacting the expression of the agouti gene. If a mother mouse—before or during pregnancy— had experienced changes in these variables, then her children would have a different distribution of fur coats and body weights from a control group who hadn't experienced these epigenetic pressures.

And some of these changes didn't just stop at the children of the mouse who was exposed. They were passed down into future generations, who continued to be affected by methylation or other epigenetic changes that had taken place generations prior.

As Whitelaw herself said, *"It changes the way we think about information transfer across generations. The mind-set at the moment is that the information we inherit from our parents is in the form of DNA. Our experiment demonstrates that it's more than just DNA you inherit. In a sense that's obvious, because what we inherit from our parents are chromosomes, and chromosomes are only 50 percent DNA. The other 50 percent is made up of protein molecules, and these proteins carry the epigenetic marks and information."*

When we inherit our parents' genes, we inherit their whole chromosomes, or the contents of those shelves—that is, their scrolls and what is written on them (the DNA), as well as some of their ribbons (methylation patterns) and other epigenetic markers. This is particularly true for the mother's epigenetics. Indeed, parts of the epigenetic code are wiped when a sperm meets an egg, but we have certain scrolls whose instructions aren't that helpful—or are even harmful—to a cell or organism's flourishing. These scrolls tend to remain heavily methylated across generations, as they aren't wiped. They maintain parental patterns of ribbons. Inherited methylation can also affect other genes near these problem scrolls, pointing to one way in which methylation can be passed down through the generations. This was the case with our agouti mice.

Rather than exposing mice to various diets or chemicals, let's now imagine that these mice made these decisions themselves. They picked the high-sugar, low-protein diet, or they nibbled on the BPA plastic. Their own behaviour led to those changes in methylation patterns, and those methylation patterns were inherited across generations, and continued to influence the expression of genes into physical characteristics.

Whose theory does that sound like? Behaviour in one generation leading to changes in the next. It's our crazy old uncle, Jean-Baptiste Lamarck, and his theory of the inheritance of acquired characteristics. Scientists in the 21st century have found potential mechanisms that align with the implications of a widely discredited 19th century theory. We are not saying that Lamarck was proved right by any means; instead, there is evidence mounting for alternate types of inheritance and evolution, rather than purely that of DNA and natural selection.

The only trouble is that this effect was observed within populations of mice, and for a specific gene with some specific characteristics. As we'll discover in an upcoming section, scientists are still trying to observe patterns of epigenetic inheritance in human populations. Objective science gets trickier and muddier when you're not allowed to control organisms' lives, force-breed them, or expose them to different levels of potentially harmful chemicals.

Over the 50 years between Crick, Watson, and Franklin (1953) discovering the double helix through the Human Genome Project (2003), genetics was the buzzword and dogma of biology and wider society. As mentioned in our introduction, it was lauded as God's code, or the language of life. Talk of histones, DNA methylation, and—less so—non-coding RNA, have only gotten much louder in the decades since, as we appreciate the importance of the interplay between genetics and all that lies beyond it: epigenetics.

From 1990 to 2000, for every published study that mentioned epigenetics, there were 100 that focused on genetics. But from 2000-2013, the number of epigenetic papers increased by more than 60 times. With more than four times the increase of 'genetic mentioning' papers over the same period, the ratio shrunk from 100:1, to less than 10:1. It seems that in scientific circles, epigenetic research—or at least that labelled as so— is on a real bull run. This suggests two things: 1) A shift in research funding towards epigenetics, meaning more people are recognising its potential, and 2) a shift in thinking and using the term *epigenetics*.

Previous seemingly unconnected research involving methylation, histones, or DMNTs, have been brought under the umbrella term of epigenetics. And as this book will tell and prove, this can be a very wide umbrella. Science is developing a system for thinking cogently about the expression of DNA, rather than simply focusing on the DNA script itself. Such a system of thinking is often referred to as a paradigm.

Darwin and Neo-Darwinian genetics have ruled the roost for more than a century now, but there is a new generation of epigenetic-focused researchers, and if they aren't calling for a change of the guard, they are at least calling for some inclusions—perhaps Conrad Waddington to sit a little higher-up on the table that Darwin still heads. For that century of Neo-Darwinism, the focus was firmly on the gene as the sole determinant of life outcomes. The fact that the latest research points the other way to more than a century of scientific inclination is exciting. Indeed, as paleobiologist Doug Erwin quipped so clearly, *"There is nothing scientists enjoy more than the prospect of a good paradigm shift."*

But all this revolutionary talk is too radical. It's not a case of toppling genetics. Instead, we need to tear open the discipline and our minds to the complex, interwoven web of effects and mechanisms that make up our cellular library. Successful theatre doesn't work with a script alone; we need actors. And actors need that script, as well as the stage notes, director's instruction, props, and costumes. It's the whole ensemble that heightens the pulse, wows the audience, and leaves them coming back for more, children in tow.

We are decoding and discovering in both genetics and epigenetics. The deeper we delve, the less distinct we find the results. The more we understand them, the less we can divide genetics and epigenetics as separate studies. Together, they form the concert of life—a concert that hopefully, having read this chapter, you will be all the more able to listen to and appreciate.

References:

https://www.tandfonline.com/doi/full/10.1080/21553769.2016.1249033

https://www.nature.com/articles/npp2012112#MOESM1

https://www.nature.com/articles/nrg.2016.83

https://www.nature.com/articles/s41419-019-1524-2#:~:text=cancer%20cells65.-,DNA%2Dbinding%20affinity,modification%20site%2C%20and%20cell%20context.

https://www.ncbi.nlm.nih.gov/pmc/articles/PMC5559844/

Youngson & Whitelaw - Transgenerational Epigentic Effects

Epigenetic inheritance at the agouti locus in the mouse - December 1999- Nature Genetics

https://genomebiology.biomedcentral.com/articles/10.1186/s13059-015-0626-0

Part Two

Epigenetics in Humans

Epigenetics

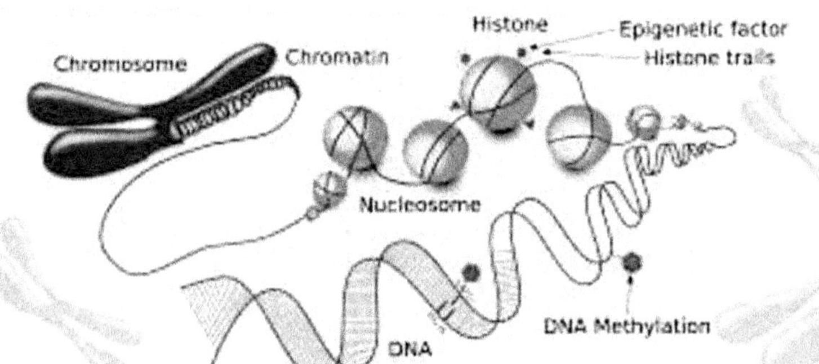

2.1

Epigenetics in Population and Between Generations - The accidental experiments of History

Human Sciences are always the fuzziest because, for many reasons, understanding the self is always trickier than understanding the external. In experiments on the self, the observer is also the subject. Clearly defined dependent and independent variables are always going to be a fantasy. On the one hand, this might apply to journeys of self-learning and spiritual insight, but it is wholly relevant to material matters like lifestyle, diet, biology, and of course, epigenetics.

In perfect laboratory experiments, we can control other variables, use the aforementioned genetically identical lab rats (mice), and, well, treat them like... lab rats. We can expose them to harmful radiation, chemicals, or feed them poor diets, and then see how it all turns out. Then, because they've only lived in a perfectly controlled lab, we can understand what caused things to turn out the way they did. Apart from a few of the more abhorrent moments of human history, we've never achieved the same laboratory conditions for humans—something we can be happy about. It's not ethically feasible to control all aspects of a human's life—sometimes purposefully introducing harmful elements—for the pursuit of scientific knowledge. This has, however, left our knowledge of human biology (and epigenetics) extremely fuzzy around the edges. For the most part, we just have to assume that humans are very similar to mice.

Thankfully though, history and reproductive biology have given us a few accidental experiments, where—by luck—most of the variables have been controlled across large enough sample populations to draw some direct learnings on how external epigenetic factors influence life outcomes. Limited by medical record-keeping, we have two examples of natural experiments with sufficient evidence: 1) the Dutch *Hongerwinter,* and 2) the Overkalix study in Sweden. And from reproductive biology, we have one consistent subgroup rich in epigenetic insight: identical twins.

Before we look at the individual, we'll look at the group. From studying epigenetics in action on populations, we can understand likely mechanisms for a given person, and from that, we can begin to optimise our individual lifestyles based on the bleeding edge of scientific research in this area.

Laboratory experiments are exceptional circumstances. War is also an example of a (hopefully) exceptional circumstance. It's partly for that reason that we look to WW2, and Netherlands under Nazi rule, for our circumstance where reality mimicked the laboratory.

In September 1944, the Nazi occupiers outlawed food and fuel transport from the South of the Netherlands to the North. The occupiers were busy shipping these goods to where the

German army needed them. As such, a country of genetically similar people, who had enjoyed plentiful food for many years, suddenly experienced an acute famine. Then, just as suddenly, at the end of the blockade, the food taps were turned on, and there was no longer a shortage. This period of malnutrition for millions was referred to as the *Hongerwinter* or Hunger Winter. In another stroke of luck, the Dutch national medical system was world-leading in many respects, and they carefully plotted the weights, heights, and health issues of their entire population throughout their years. So, what we have here is about as close as we could hope to a large-scale, genetically controlled, short-term human experiment with reliable data on the effect of malnutrition on humans. A tragedy for many humans, but a rare boon indeed for biologists.

So, what were the results of this accidental experiment?

Well, the people who were children during the Hongerwinter unsurprisingly suffered from chronic health issues. The curiosities began in the 1980s, when the children of the women who were pregnant through the troubled winter were grown adults. These 'babes of hunger' had health problems, too, having higher rates of diabetes, obesity, and mental illness than other comparable groups. We know that malnourishment in utero leads to the baby's body becoming more adapted to storing fat. Under closer inspection, methylation (the stapled ribbons or epigenetic off-switches), had occurred on the DNA that governs growth and development. Their lack of nourishment as fetuses had caused epigenetic changes, which echoed well into adult years.

Fascinatingly, there was also a difference observed depending on how the term of the pregnancy overlapped with the 6-month famine. If the pregnant mother was already six months pregnant when the famine began, the fetus was undernourished in its last few months. It was born undersize but would recover much of the initial loss, and was therefore less likely to experience health complications later on in life. However, if the mother fell pregnant halfway through the Hongerwinter and gave birth six months after it had ended, the newborn was likely to be closer to the average birth weight. However, this person was more likely to be ill throughout their lives. These findings boil down to the timing of the negative environmental stressor. If this famine happened to occur when the fetus was in its later months of development, when it gains most of its pre-birth weight, then the baby would end up smaller. But if the stressor occurred earlier in development, when the DMNT-1 library officials were still stapling their early instructions on the precious scrolls, then that critical process would have been disturbed, errors would have crept in, and the human's later life would have been blighted by the problematic coding.

The plot thickens even further. After the millennium, when the grandkids of the starving mothers, or the kids of the 'babes of hunger', were being studied, scientists found higher rates of the same health conditions. So, the initial findings indicate that certain life stressors or external conditions can impact the health outcomes across two or even three generations. David Allis, the poetic histone expert, had this to say on the matter, *"Genes cannot change an entire population in just two generations, but some memory of metabolic stress could have become heritable."* As with every respectable man of science, he also added some words of caution on what we do and do not know. Although there are some clear, specific instances of non-genetic (epigenetic) inheritance, research is still being conducted regarding what is and isn't passed between generations.

For instance, we know that if a mother loses an arm in her childhood, her children's arms will be unaffected. We know that if a woman is exposed to nuclear radiation or a chemical like Agent Orange, her children's lives will be severely affected. We now have strong evidence that if a woman is malnourished for periods of her life, her children will also likely be affected. However, the question of whether mental stress, levels of exercise, types of diet, traumas, and quality of relationships can lead to situations where epigenetic material is passed from one generation to another is still up for debate. There is growing research and experimental evidence on (relatively similar) mammals, suggesting that more and more of these factors are relevant across multiple generations. Whether these environmental factors affect our own epigenetics— impacting our own lives—is a more settled case. The mounting evidence affirms that they do. We can be sure that our choices affect the expression of our otherwise fixed DNA, and we have good reason to believe that our choices impact the expressions of our children's DNA, as well.

Let's look across the Baltic Sea to Sweden, and specifically to a little-known northerly province called Överkalix. We can thank the wonderfully detailed and comprehensive record keeping of 19th century Swedes, and the relative isolation of the municipality, for this natural experiment. The sample group is quite smaller than the millions affected in the Hongerwinter. This accidental experiment included 303 adults, and 1,818 children and grandchildren, with detailed historical records starting in 1890, and ending in 1995. We have data on people's health outcomes, as well as on harvests and food prices, which acts as a proxy for food availability.

Various intergenerational effects were observed. Of particular interest were the ones passed down by men and fathers. The sons of early-smoking fathers had greater BMIs yet the same effect was not significant for daughters. Moreover, if the grandfather had been exposed to periods of feast and famine, then the grandson was more likely to have heart problems yet, once more, the granddaughter was seemingly unaffected. The granddaughter's heart health was only affected by her grandmother's malnourishment. Outcomes from mothers to children tend to be easier to find than those from fathers to children, which is one of the reasons why Överkalix is so powerful: effects were observed from the paternal side *and* the maternal one.

This is important. True epigenetic inheritance occurs when the methylation or histone patterns are passed from one generation's DNA directly to another's. This is called *parental imprinting.* Those scientists who deny parental imprinting instead claim that the environment of the womb of an unhealthy woman will cause epigenetic changes in the fetus through development, rather than epigenetic patterns being directly copied across genetic material. Beyond this, there is also a case that when a pregnant woman is exposed to an external stressor, which has the power to alter epigenetics, then the stressor can be passed down to three generations. The first generation is clearly the mother herself, the second generation is the fetus in her womb, and the third generation is the prospective grandchild, who is essentially formed from the reproductive cells developing in the genitals of the fetus. Thus, we can argue that one external stressor might directly influence three sets of epigenetics, without the mechanism of parental imprinting. Observing the effect in the 4th generation would incontrovertibly prove epigenetic inheritance has occurred.

The scientists who deny parental imprinting in humans have more ground to stand on when discussing effects from mothers, but the fetus doesn't grow up inside the father. There's one shot of DNA in the semen, and that's it. So, if we can observe what looks to be epigenetic inheritance through the father's line, then we can be certain that we aren't seeing environmental factors of the womb. We've got many instances of this in lab rats, but Överkalix was one of the first times we could prove this in humans. True, we only recognise parental imprinting in 1-2% of human genes, but we still have instances of it occurring and are finding more data points day by day.

The evidence is still emerging, but if found to be significant, then we have a case where your grandmother's diet and lifestyle affects you, and in turn, your diet and lifestyle affects your grandkids.

How does that knowledge affect the way we live?

Well, opportunity and danger are two sides of the same coin. Where some might see their bad lifestyle choices plaguing their progeny, others may see their determination and virtue benefiting those who come after them. One glass is half-empty, focusing on the damage we might do, while the other is half-full, emphasising the epigenetic gifts we might bestow.

Despite the view you adopt, one thing is certain: With this knowledge, the stakes are higher. Your life choices may well affect you the most, but it doesn't stop there. Your actions will ripple across generations.

And with that in mind, this book just became that much more essential. We'll get to the modern scientific advice at the end of this section, and in the next section, we'll look at the ancient wisdom that was aimed to aid us in the same way.

Twins and Epigenetics - Diverging Double Trouble

If diamonds are a girl's best friend, then identical twins are a geneticist's best friends. Twins are one of those human experiments that nature provided to us, without us having to get into ethically dodgy places. Studying identical twins can give us insight into the balance of nature and nurture, or—as we can now call it—genetics and epigenetics.

Identical twins occur when the *zygote*, the fertilised egg, splits into two zygotes. Since both zygotes came from the same egg and same sperm, the zygotes are genetically and epigenetically identical. When the twins are born—let's call them Lara and Lyra—the babies are still genetically identical, but they will be, ever so slightly, epigenetically different. This is because they will have minutely different experiences and nutrient exposures in the womb, which are likely to cause very small divergences in the behaviour of their library officials and in the precise rolling of the scrolls on their shelves.

Then, as the twins grow up, they will have differing lifestyles. Let's say Lara is more active as a toddler and loves to run up and down the garden. Lyra eats all of her vegetables, but Lara only eats chips and meat. There are some differences in their environment and lifestyle, but really, they live in the same house, and are fed similar things. Their epigenetic situations will be more divergent than when they were born, but there won't be large differences.

Then, as life gets more complex, Lyra puts a great deal of stress on herself in trying to be perfect in her schoolwork and in her relationships. Lara, on the other hand, is very laid back; nothing seems to faze her. Lara learns to enjoy lots of beer and starts smoking, but Lyra only has a very occasional glass of red wine. Lyra starts work as a machine engineer in a chemical factory, whereas Lara loves the great outdoors and works as a lumberjack. Lara takes up meditation and yoga, whereas Lyra takes up a Xanax prescription to manage her stress. Soon, their lifestyles, experiences, and exposures start to differ dramatically, and we should be able to find significantly different methylation and histone patterns within the nuclei of their cells. Now, with the wondrous technical advances in genetics and epigenetic coding discussed in the past section, we have the techniques and equipment to observe and track specific methylation and histone pattern differences in real time, throughout their lives. It's these same epigenetic differences in their cells that will have an impact on their health, mentality, and lifestyle. The differences inside the nuclei will cause differences in their lives. And as we've discussed in this chapter, it may also cause differences in the lives of their children, and possibly even grandchildren.

These emerging epigenetic differences can cause the lives, preferences, and health of otherwise genetically identical twins to differ more prominently than those of distant cousins. These are non-trivial life-and-death matters, like the likelihood of cancer or heart and mental diseases occurring. What is so wondrous about twins from a scientist's standpoint is that we can observe this fascinating experiment of starting at the exact same point, and ending apart, to build a picture of how lifestyle choices affect life outcomes. But even more than that, we can look at the prevalence of different diseases amongst identical twins and fraternal twins, discerning how important genetics are compared to our environment regarding occurrences of health issues.

Since we can assume that the living environments of fraternal twins and identical twins are likely to be similar, when there is a disease or trait that identical twins are likely to share, then we can safely assume that's a condition predominantly driven by genetics. Conversely, when there is a disease that one twin may experience whereas the other may not—and isn't more likely to experience it than fraternal twins are—then we can safely assume that disease is driven more by the environment, or epigenetic factors. See the graph below of condition rates between twins of both kinds.

This is important for us to understand from a standpoint of improving our environment so that we can ultimately improve our epigenetics and our life outcomes. The conditions to the left of this graph may be trickier to reduce the probability of through lifestyle choices and changing living conditions. However, the health issues down the scale on the right are clearly ones we can significantly impact through our own behaviour and decisions. Those most within our control are also those that most afflict our society, including hypertension, diabetes, cancer, stroke, and arthritis. The way you understand this concept really depends on whether you perceive the glass to be half empty or half full. Let's illustrate this in a more creative manner, shifting away from scientific terms for just a moment.

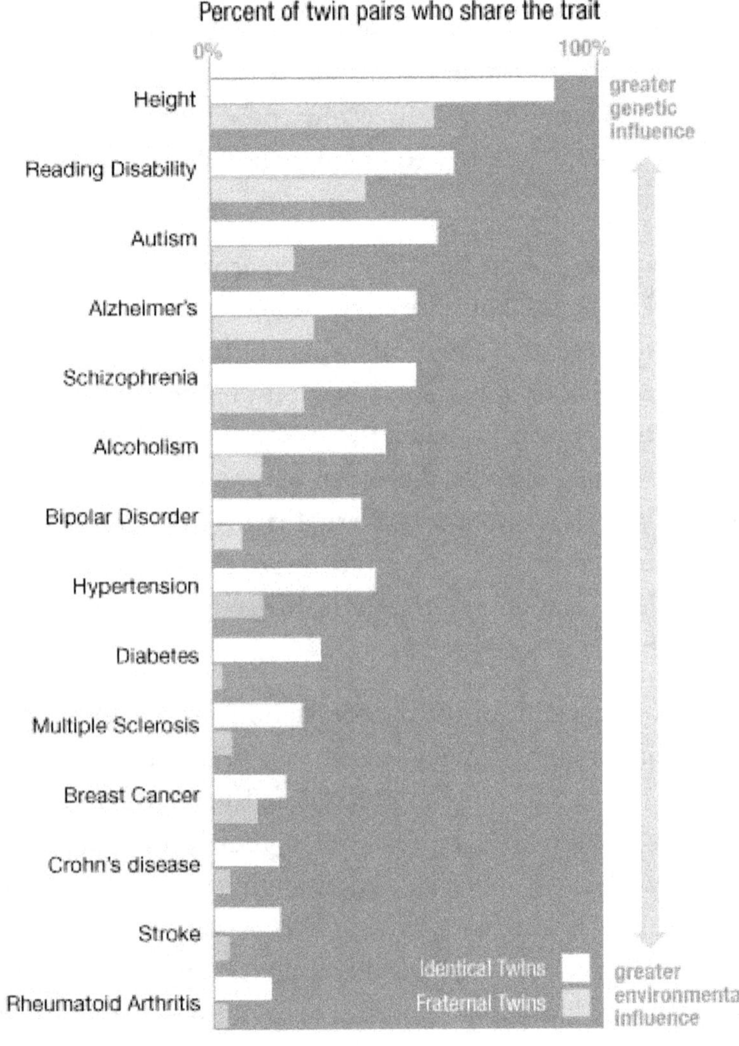

[5]

____

5 Source: https://learn.genetics.utah.edu/content/epigenetics/twins

Winnie the Pooh's Eeyore would point out how our living and environmental conditions are so poor that the diseases people in the developed world suffer from most are all epigenetically driven: *"Don't we live in such a toxic and unhealthy state?"*

But Tigger would posit something entirely different. If these are the most widespread diseases that cause the most pain and suffering in our world, then aren't we lucky because we have the power to lessen how often we suffer from them? *"What an opportunity for improvement,"* he'd say.

Over the remaining pages of this book, we will adopt a smidge of Eeyore's view to identify the toxic elements of our lives that cause these problems. But really, this is Tigger's book. We focus on how we can avoid those toxic elements to improve our odds, and more crucially, determine which therapies are out there to repair the epigenetic damage we've already done. In progressing through this lifework—this healing path—we will create a better live for ourselves, handing over the best epigenome we can to our descendants. They will need it more than ever, as they also inherit our Earth.

2.3

___

Scientific Theories to Real World Methods: A Cautionary Tale

It's important to re-emphasise how cutting-edge and exploratory the kind of research that delves into epigenetic mechanisms really is. In the first section of this book, we mentioned how scientists have only just recently—in the last 18 months—developed a technique to see the bricks in the wall of the libraries that are our cells' nuclei. And in a sense, the whole history of genetic understanding has been a history of magnification. This first started with Robert Hooke in 1665 when he first used the microscope on a piece of cork bark to discover the cell. Then, in 1835, Robert Brown got closer and found the nucleus. In 1953, Watson, Crick, and Franklin discovered the shape of the DNA chromosome. In 2003, the Human Genome Project was completed, and we had zoomed down into the level of base pairs within DNA. Now, in the 2020s, we are looking at methylation—the hangers on the chromosome's base pair. And with each consequent level of magnification, we are better understanding the mechanics of organic life.

However, some things can only be discovered by zooming out and looking at whole organisms—or populations of organisms, for that matter. We can't understand how a human and her children are affected by malnourishment only through looking at their chromosomes. We need to study their lives, alongside the lives of many others within an effective sample group. We can only start to progress in understanding when we partner discoveries on a large scale with the lessons learned on the smallest scales we have access to. When we've examined the above and below, we can find applicable theories, putting them into practice to improve our lives. This chapter focuses on just that. From a base of scientific knowledge, what can we as individuals do to improve our epigenetics to heal our bodies and minds?

Before we use the latest base of scientific knowledge to find these answers, it's also informative to look to the past, back to when we had a lower level of scientific knowledge. This can help us understand how those earlier theories led us to certain methods and practices, some of which still stand-up today, whilst other more damaging ones have thankfully been well-consigned to history's dustbin. We will cover the ancient's indirect understanding of epigenetics in Part three of this book, but for now, let's examine the good and bad of the last 150 years of theorising on human health and its environment.

1859 saw the publication of Charles Darwin's origin of species, where he explored and expounded the process of natural selection in driving evolution in animals. There's one fascinating omission in this book: us. He didn't tackle the subject of humans, probably because he knew it would attract enough debate and uproar. That's why in 1871, he went on to publish his second most famous book: *The Descent of Man, and Selection in Relation to Sex*. Right from the title, we can identify that this book focuses on humans, our close relation to animals, and how we were also subject to the laws of evolution. This was a fairly grand leap in a society where many thought the world and all its contents had been created less than 10,000 years prior, and where humans were seen as divinely designed guardians of the Earth, separate from animals.

As we know from Part 1, there were two major competing schools of evolution in the 19th century: Darwinism and Lamarckism. Both were based on the idea that an organism's environment influences its evolution, albeit through two different mechanisms: 1) Natural selection of mutated characteristics and 2) Inheritance of acquired characteristics. So, with these two points in mind, contemporary thinkers understood that evolution depends on environment, and that evolution applies to humans, thus concluding that our environment determines our evolution.

Related to this was research into the origins of mankind. Darwin, amongst others, believed in monogenesis, meaning a human ancestor had emerged in one place (likely Africa) and had travelled and populated the world. Environmental factors like climate and diet led to the divergence of physical traits in humankind—our size, our skin colour, our bone and muscle composition, and so on. This was one school of thought in Race Theory, in which the belief was that environmental factors had caused differences in human evolution.

Scientists now and scientists then would agree that evolution equates to change. But whether that change is good or bad is subjective, and, suddenly we have disagreements. From the objective, scientific standpoint, there is no positive or negative evolution; there is only change to adapt to a shift in environmental factors. Some birds on remote islands lost their ability to fly because there were no predators in their environment, so they no longer needed to fly to survive. This is neither good nor bad. However, some would argue that these birds have lost a key and defining attribute. Some would say they have devolved due to a lack of evolutionary pressure. After the great leaps forward in biological thinking in the 19th century, it didn't take long for some to apply the same analysis to humankind: With poor environmental factors or a lack of sufficient competition, humans too might also devolve. Their conclusion: At one point, the human species was at risk of degeneration.

Most people exposed to these evolutionary ideas were white, male, and rich Western intellectuals, who believed that most people of different colours and classes were separate and other to them. Many of these thinkers saw these 'others' as a different group, race, or species, and usually, as somehow lower, less civilised, or less evolved. Hence, in their minds, the risk of degeneration of the human species meant that, in essence, there would be fewer 'great people like them' in the future, and more 'bad people'. This 'terrible future' could happen in two ways. First, the 'other people' have more children than the 'like people', and so, the population balance changes; or second, 'like people' living in poor environments would degenerate into 'other people'.

This dichotomy relates to the central toss-up of nature versus nurture that we've discussed thus far. The first 'road to hell' represents nature, where worse quality DNA proliferates through the many children of the 'other people', whilst the best DNA is limited to the few children of the 'like people'—traits are fixed and inherited; you have good blood or bad blood and that's it. The second option is nurture, where environmental factors help determine the qualities of your person and their DNA—the environment that someone is raised in determines their outcome. Throughout the 20th century, different groups in different countries explored both of these paths with wildly differing results. However, they all had the same aim: To improve mankind.

First, let's briefly review outcomes of the school of nature. Francis Galton, the 19th century English polymath, used his understanding of statistics and genetic inheritance to study geniuses and illnesses. He looked at dynasties of brilliant artists, musicians, and philosophers, and compared them with families of the mentally or physically ill, or those with substance abuse problems. He found what he saw as statistical proof for inherited abilities and disabilities in humans. He also coined the term *eugenics*, meaning 'well-born' or 'from good genes'. He saw potential in mankind for breeding in positive attributes, and breeding out problematic ones. He also left a warning: *"Over-zeal leading to hasty action would do harm by holding out expectations of a near golden age which would certainly be falsified and cause the science ["eugenics"] to be discredited."*

Different political groups around the world looked to apply eugenics as a guard against what they considered degeneration. This led to sterilisation laws and other inhumane eugenic practices across the USA, Europe, and other countries around the world. These laws sought to prevent the 'other people'— which referred to different groups—from reproducing and 'worsening' the evolutionary balance in the population. Although many of the theorists and early legislation had their origins in the USA, the UK, and Nordic countries, the most extreme, famous, and terrible example of applied eugenic thought was the Third Reich of Nazi Germany. If the hateful ideas were imported from abroad, they matured fully in Germany, where the eugenic cleansing of Jews, Gypsies, Slavic people, gays, and Black people was structured as perhaps the central objective and purpose of society. We are all aware of the horrors, trauma, and pain that resulted from this application of supposedly scientific theory to the real world.

Eugenics became totally associated with that toxicity, and consequently, was discredited in the post-war years. Galton's prophetic warning of someone applying eugenics with "over-zeal" advertising "a near golden age" neatly fits onto Hitler proclaiming a utopic *Thousand-Year Reich* with his *Final Solution*. Given how eugenics was applied in Germany and other countries, it has understandably—and arguably correctly—been consigned to history's dustbin as dangerous pseudoscience in the 20th century.

Now, let's approach the second side: nurture. The concern in the discussion regarding human evolution and degeneration was that poor environments would produce poor humans. The 18th and 19th centuries in Western Europe were the era of the Industrial Revolution and great urbanisation. In a very short period, poor people from around the countryside were now tightly packed into cities, and working long hours in difficult and dangerous jobs, far away from the farms that grew fresh food. Karl Marx saw the creation of the proletariat, whereas other scientific contemporaries viewed it as the start of the degeneration of mankind. An avalanche of social and health problems arrived with this shift, including an increase in diseases like cholera, smallpox, typhus, sexually transmitted diseases, and tuberculosis. This change also came with an increase in crime, alcoholism, prostitution, vagrancy, child beggars, and violence, as well as other mental and physical disorders. Many observers at the time saw these problems as emerging from human degeneration, with the belief that people were getting worse in all respects.[6]

If the eugenic solution was to prevent as many of these people from procreating, the other, more liberal solution was to improve the environment, thus improving the people, as well. This was a brand of social Darwinism, and was associated with social hygiene and welfare. There were calls for the abolition of urban slums for improved suburban housing, the growing of fresh vegetables in city allotments, and even rural holidays for urban populations. The social campaigners believed that a reconnection to the countryside and to a more natural way of living would improve the lives and health outcomes of the new urban proletariat.

Industrial millionaires on both sides of the Atlantic were also often central to these efforts. In America, Andrew Carnegie and John D. Rockefeller gave—in combination—almost a billion dollars (which would be the equivalent of tens of billions in

---

6 British society found the empirical proof of this degeneration in the poor military performance in the Second Boer War in 1899. The soldiers and recruits were seen to be in such poor physical condition that "the Great British Army could be beaten by a rabble of South African farmers." Consequently, in 1903, an Inter-Departmental Committee on Physical Deterioration was set up to uncover the true roots of the problem. Interestingly enough for us, they found "abundant signs of physical defect traceable to neglect, poverty, and ignorance, but it is not possible to obtain any satisfactory or conclusive evidence of hereditary physical deterioration." In essence, the problem with the people was in their living environment, rather than in their genes.

today's money) to various institutions promoting health and education. Rockefeller founded the Rockefeller Sanitary Commission in 1909, which eradicated hookworm, whilst Carnegie was known as the 'patron saint' of the public library. Intriguingly, Rockefeller also gave funds for eugenic research to Eugene Fischer in the Kaiser's Germany, who would go on to be a 'scientific architect' of Hitler's Final Solution. In the UK, there was the Rowntree industrial family. After making his millions in food manufacturing, Joseph Rowntree set up a foundation (still operating today) to investigate the root causes of social problems. He also built a village, New Earswick, as a model in how to provide decent living conditions for industrial workers. His son, Seebohm Rowntree, was a pioneering researcher into poverty and improving social welfare. Private philanthropy led the way initially, but over time, the UK government integrated the same social health and hygiene movement into the Beveridge report, which led to the creation of the National Health Service in 1948—the first health system in any Western society to offer free medical care to the entire population.

So, this was the other approach designed to improve the stock of humans in society, through improving the diet and living environment of the people who were experiencing problems. Here, we have a fascinating case study of a combination of scientific discoveries regarding evolutionary and human biology leading to two wildly different applications in the real world with very different results and legacies. One approach was built on a primitive understanding of genetics, while the other was built on an equally primitive understanding of epigenetics. The nature-genetic approach stated that peoples' qualities were fixed, while the nurture-epigenetics principle was that qualities were changeable depending on the environment. In this case study, the genetic approach of the Nazis led to the sterilisation and termination of millions of Jews and other peoples. On the other hand, the epigenetic approach of social campaigners and philanthropists led to public health and education, social welfare, and housing.

Conrad Waddington, the father of epigenetics, was fervently anti-Nazi and a Marxist. Marxism holds that the changing conditions will lead humans (the proletariat) to a better society for the collective good. As such, it fits well that his ideas empowered us to think that people's qualities and lives could be bettered by improving their environments. A Jew, poor person, gypsy, or any other sort of person are not fixed by a predetermined genetic destiny. Their living conditions and life choices will have a major impact on their life outcomes.

This is one of the great powers and weaknesses of science. Scientific research is meant to be objective, beyond morals of what should and shouldn't be. It's then up to non-scientists, politicians, campaigners, and every day people to decide how to interpret the science, and which intentions to place behind it. In this case, the idea that genetic qualities were fixed led to monumental human tragedies, whilst the power of the environment and what would be termed as epigenetics allowed for great leaps forward in our collective humanity. The rest of this book rests firmly on the latter approach, believing that people's destinies are not determined by their start—genetic or otherwise. Instead, it can all be chalked up to the way we live life, the choices we make, and the approaches we take. And so, it's all the more important that we are well-informed by the most cutting edge science and the most ancient wisdom on how to live life free of physical, mental, or spiritual illness.

2.4

———

Modern Epigenetics in Practice -
Diets from the Data

Most of the advances in social welfare to stave off supposed threats of degeneration were all conceived and carried out in a time when the hard science of modern epigenetics still remained hidden. In one way or another, humans always had some understanding of how environment, diet, and living conditions could lead to either disease or good health; but until the second half of the 20th century, and more so since the millennium, we had no conception of the fundamental dynamics in how these factors can change the way in which our body lives and breathes, how our heart beats, and how our mind fires.

Although the modern science of epigenetics is still in its infancy, it has changed that belief. And similar to Galton's warning of eugenics, it's vital that we approach epigenetics in the correct way so that humans can harness its potential for good. It's crucial that we don't leap to hypotheses that might do damage or destabilise epigenetic progress in genuine areas. After all, you don't run before you can walk. Most of all, it's vital that the intentions behind applied epigenetics are rooted in the individual and collective good. As with most scientific developments, within epigenetics, there is the potential for commercialisation, weaponization, or restriction of universal access.

Now starts the book's sections we've all been waiting for. We start by asking the questions that likely led you here in the first place: How should I live? What should I eat? What habits should I heal to maintain good health, and to live well by my epigenetics?

We'll start with the positives—the areas that scientists have observed that can do more of to improve your functional epigenome. The most researched and possibly most powerful aspect of this is diet, so let's start there.

The old adage, "You are what you eat," is given a new meaning when examined through an epigenetic lens. There are foods, cooking methods, and cooking utensils that are now being proven as instrumental in altering your epigenome over the course of your life. There are now a number of studies that both prove and directly explain how natural compounds found in foods can help in cell regulation and disease prevention.

In looking at the diet and the epigenome, cancer is a very powerful place to begin because it is a sure-fire way to recognise that cells have ceased to function in the normal way. That is, things have happened, or damage has been done, that affects the way in which the cell operates. Since the normal operation is driven by instructions from the library, we can conclude that something is likely awry in the library operations department. Scientists have found that when our DNMTs—our ribbon-stapling library officials—change their behaviour, numerous diseases come about, including autism, cardiovascular diseases, obesity, and Type-2 diabetes, as well as cancer.

As more and more research is being completed, the role epigenetics plays in these diseases is being uncovered, and we are attributing increased importance to it. However, this swings both positively and negatively. Scientists are finding ever more causal links between these diseases and exposure to various drugs, chemicals used in pesticides, environmental compounds, and inorganic contaminants. In fact, scientists are starting to trace the ways in which consuming these problematic chemicals—even in incredibly small doses—can alter the work of those library officials, thus causing abnormalities. That's the bad news. The good news is in how they are also finding the power of diet in either preventing or repairing those abnormalities. In animal research, animals who had a diet deficient in folate, choline, and methionine (compounds found in plants), all experienced a change in the DNA methylation patterns of their liver; cancer had also developed there.[7] Changing the diet to one full of these important compounds reversed some of the methylation, and in many cases, prevented the cancer from occurring in the first place.

These plant compounds are called *phytochemicals* in science-speak. They underpin a lot of epigenetic dietary research. Their epigenetic uses vary. Some are involved in methionine synthesis—they are the raw materials that the ribbons are made of—while some help our cells clean themselves after ribbons (methyls) are made. Others, yet again, are involved with histone acetylation—the post-it notes (acetyls) pasted on the spools

---

7 70. Poirier LA. Methyl group deficiency in hepatocarcinogenesis. Drug Metab Rev. 1994;26(1–2):185–199.

(histones). Think about these nutrients as the supply depot for our library department. If you give our officials the best equipment, you stand the best chance of optimal operational performance.

Before we get into some of the individual highlights, below is a table outlining some of the key phytochemicals and dietary compounds, which are lighting up epigenetic research. The table also lists which foods you can get them from:

Nutrient	Food Origin	Epigenetic Role
Methionine	Sesame seeds, Brazil nuts, fish, peppers, spinach	SAM synthesis
Folic Acid	Leafy vegetables, sunflower seeds, baker's yeast, liver	Methionine synthesis
Vitamin B12	Meat, liver, shellfish, milk	Methionine synthesis
Vitamin B6	Meats, whole grain products, vegetables, nuts	Methionine synthesis
SAM-e (SAM)	Popular dietary supplement pill; unstable in food	Enzymes transfer methyl groups from SAM directly to the DNA
Choline	Egg yolks, liver, soy, cooked beef, chicken, veal, and turkey	Methyl donor to SAM
Betaine	Wheat, spinach, shellfish, and sugar beets	Break down the toxic by-products of SAM synthesis
Resveratrol	Red wine	Removes acetyl groups from histones, improving health (shown in lab mice)
Genistein	Soy, soy products	Increased methylation, cancer prevention, unknown mechanism

Sulforaphane	Broccoli	Increased histone acetylation turning on anti-cancer genes
Butyrate	A compound produced in the intestine when dietary fibre is fermented	Increased histone acetylation turning on 'protective' genes, increased lifespan (shown in the lab in flies)
Diallyl sulphide (DADS)	Garlic	Increased histone acetylation turning on anti-cancer genes

As with many endeavours, it's best to start our tour of epigenetic eats with a nice cup of tea—the most consumed beverage worldwide, with more than three billion cups consumed daily. The three most common types of tea are black, green, and oolong. Many teas are rich in polyphenols, which are compounds found in fruit and vegetables that have a range of epigenetic functions. They can help in remodelling chromatin (the shelves), activating good genes that have been silenced, prohibiting DMNTs from partaking in certain bad behaviours, and rearranging histones. Polyphenols' range of function make them powerful partners in putting together positive epigenetic diets.

In fact, various mechanisms have been identified that help explain the preventive nature of polyphenols, including their ability to alter the epigenome in cancer cells by chromatin remodelling or by reactivating silenced genes [76–78]. The chemo-preventative potential of dietary polyphenols can be traced to their ability to inhibit DNMTs, as well as their ability to act as histone modifiers. Both properties of dietary polyphenols can significantly change the epigenome of cancer cells, and are viewed as attractive possibilities for anticancer therapeutics. Catechins are particularly abundant in green tea.

They are a type of polyphenol that are especially epigenetically powerful. Epigallocatechin gallate (EGCG) is the most efficient of the catechins, and accounts for more than 50% of the active compounds in green tea. A range of studies have found positive correlations between consuming EGCG and lower incidences of breast, prostate, skin, ovarian, and a range of other cancers.

Before we get into solid foods, let's linger a little longer in the drink's cabinet. The polyphenol resveratrol is found in peanuts, cranberries, and blueberries, though it is most concentrated in grapes' skin, and so, in red wine, as well. It has antioxidant and anti-inflammatory properties. Resveratrol impacts the growth and division of cells, thus controlling the creation and spread of cancer in this manner. When cancerous mice were given resveratrol, it improved the state of their existing cancers and increased their survival rate. There are various mechanisms reviewed for this, most of them involving DMNTs and certain genes, which suppress tumour growth. So, don't feel guilty for having a glass of red wine here and there; your epigenetics will thank you.

Now, let's examine the spice cabinet. Turmeric has been a mainstay of Indian and Chinese medicine for millennia, with curcumin being the main and active ingredient. Here is an example of ancient societies recognising epigenetic outcomes, without directly understanding the mechanisms involved. Curcumin affects DMNT behaviour and methylation patterns, while also acting on both sides of the post-it note equation. Histone acetyltransferases (HATs) are enzymes that help in putting post-it notes on spools (acetylation). Histone deacetylases (HDACs) are enzymes that do the opposite, working toward taking off the post-it notes. When histones have lots of post-it notes, the spools become more spread out. When there are a few post-it notes, the spools are tightly packed against one another. As we mentioned earlier, loosely packed scrolls can be easily read and copied, but less so for tightly packed ones. What is so interesting about curcumin is that it's one of the few polyphenols that can, in some cases, stop HAT enzymes, and in others, stop HDAC enzymes. Curcumin can act like a referee, blowing its whistle when either side of the opposing players does something wrong. To get the most out of curcumin, it's best sprinkled over your morning eggs, or mixed in with soy sauce, as the phosphatidylcholine makes it more available for your body to absorb.

Your humble but ubiquitous garlic clove is another candidate for an epigenetic diet. Garlic wards off evil, demons, and vampires in various cultures and tales from around the world. You just need to translate the symbols into reality, swapping demons for diseases. Garlic has a healthy complex of compounds, including Vitamins A, B, C, E, free amino acids, organosulfur, and selenium. Garlic acts to slow down cell cycles and lower cell death, slow down the creation of new blood vessels, and modify our histones. It may be bad for your breath, but the long-held wisdom and newly minted science that supports cooking with lots of garlic cannot be refuted.

The school ground saying goes as follows, "Beans, beans! Good for the heart. The more you eat, the more you fart!" At least the first part of this can be backed up by epigenetic research. Flavonoids are the most common class of polyphenols. There are six different flavonoid types, and they are found in a whole range of plants, from onions, to cacao, to broccoli, and to grapefruit. One of the most well-studied flavonoid types is isoflavones. They are often found in beans—fava, mung, or green. Isoflavones are most concentrated in soybeans, specifically as the compound genistein. Genistein targets several types of cancer, likely through histone acetylation and DNA methylation. It is also the other known referee for HATs and HDACs like curcumin. Human research on genistei's impact is also crucial to explore. Healthy women were given low or high doses of isoflavones daily through a menstrual cycle. The study found that a high intake of genistein led to the silencing (methylation) of five genes that are active in breast cancer. Genistein was seen to act in a similar way to oestrogen and is often referred to as *phytoestrogen* (plant oestrogen). Don't think to get your genistein through soy sauce. Consuming enough in that form would be difficult, and would overload your body with salt. It's better to turn to tofu, tempeh, or even fresh soybeans.

Finally, let's turn to some of the vegetables that may account for the backbone of your meal. Isothiocyanates are a phytochemical found in cruciferous vegetables like broccoli. Isothiocyanates are powerful in speeding up the death of problematic cells and in preventing those cells from proliferating, as was discovered in a study that examined tumours in rats. Isothiocyanate was also found to increase histone acetylation in mouse leukaemia cells. In humans, broccoli sprouts were seen to be effective in controlling HDAC activity—taking off the post-it notes that make problematic genes more tightly wound and less often read. Beyond isothiocyanates, cruciferous vegetables are also excellent sources of folates. Folic acid, or natural folates, have long been recommended supplements in the diets of pregnant and nursing mothers. They are vital across a wide range of areas of human development. We are now also recognising their role in maintaining and developing health, as folate helps regulate the biosynthesis, repair, and methylation of DNA. A lack of folates can lead to multiple diseases and health issues. So, try to consume cruciferous vegetables like cabbage, cauliflower, and Brussels sprouts, and keep lots of room for broccoli, as well.

So, we've looked at the epigenetics of some individual ingredients, but what about whole diet types? The Mediterranean Diet has received the most attention from a healthy-ageing perspective. The NU-AGE study led the way with a one-year experiment that observed 120 elderly people, 60 of whom were from Italy, and 60 of whom were from Poland. Both groups were fed the same Mediterranean diet. The Italians were the control group, and had been following this particular diet for their whole lives. The Polish were the test group, who had not previously eaten this way on a consistent basis. The test variable was Horvath's clock, which is an epigenetic measure of age. It effectively measures how many important CPG island gene sequences are methylated. A young person should have very few, and an old person will have more as library officials make more mistakes over time. The results of the study demonstrated that the Mediterranean Diet was especially significant in reducing the epigenetic age of Polish females, particularly those who were older at the time the study had begun. Polish men also showed some improvement, with specific effects observed in metabolism, cell cycle regulation, and immunity from disease. These changes were all a result of adopting a new diet for one year, leaving all other lifestyle aspects constant, in people who had been following a different diet for 60 years or more.

The final section of this book will dive deeper into exercises and epigenetics in practical application, but it's important to note that exercise also has a significant effect on our epigenome. It's a topic that we are still decoding, and still researching. In an interesting Swedish study conducted in 2014, scientists asked 23 people to bicycle using just one leg for 45 minutes a day over the course of three months. They then compared the muscle cells of both legs, before and after the experiment. They found that in the bicycled leg, new epigenetic patterns had developed, which were associated with insulin response, inflammation, and energy metabolism. In short, the exercise had triggered a functional improvement in the epigenome of that specific leg. Beyond these changes to the stationary cells in the body, scientists have also observed that even after 20-minute bouts of intense exercise, we experience a boost in our immune system from miRNA's altering gene expression in our white blood cells. This was significant after a single bout of exercise, further emphasising the importance of implementing daily movement into our lives.

Now, let's have a brief look at some of the negatives—that is, life's threats to your epigenome. We won't spend too long on this topic, but just as it's important to understand how to live, it's also important to understand how *not* to live. In the battle for the body, let's take a leaf out of Sun Tzu's the Art of War and, "*Know thy enemy.*"

We can start with the opposite of exercise, which is a sedentary lifestyle, and its usual partner in crime: obesity. These are risk factors for just about all the illnesses that afflict our modern societies. You can determine whether someone is obese simply be examining the methylation patterns on the genes that regulate metabolism, inflammation, and insulin sensitivity. Eating less and exercising more will lead to a caloric deficit, but specific epigenetic interventions (in diet or elsewhere) may enable more rapid improvement, as we start to rewrite the problematic patterns of ribbons and post-it notes. What is more encouraging is that we can recognise that certain (rare) people have a strong genetic predisposition to obesity, but their destiny is not fixed to being fat. Again, through specific epigenetically targeted nutrition, methylation patterns can be altered back into their favour.

What about the other legal substances that we (rather unsuccessfully) prohibit our children from using, such as alcohol and tobacco? It's not new information that tobacco smoke is carcinogenic, causing inflammation through the body, and the thickening of artery walls. Benzopyrene, a major chemical in cigarettes responsible for many of the habit's ills, did not affect DNA methylation in the lungs in trials.[8] However, cigarette smoke was seen to decrease important histone modifications in lung tissue cells, similar to the changes found in lung cancer patients. Also, problematically low levels of methylation have been found in the white blood cells of lung cancer patients who also smoke.[9] There have also been studies conducted on young children who were exposed to smoke in their mother's womb. This exposure changed methylation patterns on the important CPG islands on eight genes that are crucial for normal development, and are common across most mammals. The same effect was observed in an experiment on rats, proving that normal gene expression resumed one week

---

8 Tommasi S, Kim Si, Zhong X, Wu X, Pfeifer Gp, Besaratinia A. Investigating the epigenetic effects of a prototype smoke-derived carcinogen in human cells. PLoS One. 2010;5(5):e10594.
9 Woodson K, Mason J, Choi Sw, et al. Hypomethylation of p53 in peripheral blood DNA is associated with the development of lung cancer. Cancer Epidemiol Biomarkers Prev. 2001;10(1):69–74.

after the cessation of smoke exposure.[10] That's not to say that this healing effect carries into humans, but it gives a little hope in an otherwise dire situation.

Now, onto the liquid vice of our society: booze. Unlike tobacco, ethyl alcohol doesn't change the expression of genes by itself. Instead, it changes the impact of other epigenetically active substances. And so, in its effect towards cancer, it's known as a co-carcinogen. There have been studies to suggest that it impacts the role of folate in methylation, as well as alcohol in conjunction with Vitamin B6 in increasing colon cancer. There is also slowly growing evidence that alcohol intake can lead to low methylation in blood cells. When it comes to brain development and damage, the effects of alcohol are clearer: There are clear negative effects on our epigenome concerning growth and the brain, which are directly attributable to alcohol. These have been proven in a wide range of studies on mice, and beyond this, we have many unfortunate human examples of this that we've developed from observing the children of alcoholic mothers. There has been less research on the specific epigenetic impact of ongoing alcohol consumption in adults; however, indications are strong here for an epigenetic (co) action of excess alcohol.

In sum, very moderate consumption of red wine is likely more helpful than harmful through the good effects of resveratrol and other polyphenols. But as we know, moderation in drinks is a very fine line indeed, and one that we usually trespass. For some, it may just be easier to cut booze out entirely, putting

____

10Izzotti A, Larghero P, Longobardi M, et al. Dose-responsiveness and persistence of microRNA expression alterations induced by cigarette smoke in mouse lung. Mutat Res. 2010 to bed any neurological epigenetic risks, and relying on dark fruits and berries for those polyphenol complexes. For others, cutting out alcohol may not be so feasible. In those cases, quality over quantity should be the adage. Be reassured that the epigenetic effect of alcohol is not direct in nature; it's a partner in crime. And so, being aware of epigenetic living in other respects and adopting healthy habits can mediate some of its negative effects.

Now, we can move beyond the things that we purposefully consume, and shift to things that get into our system through our lived environment. It's easier when we have some agency over our food, drinks, and exercise, but environmental pollutants are ever-present in our public water, in the products we use to clean our house, in the fuels we use for transport and heat, and in the chemicals we use to grow our food. The level of research required to be aware of these pollutants and to recognise their sources in our lives is vast and complex. But understanding this is only half the struggle. It requires an even greater effort to live in our modern world, with its conveniences and customs, and yet find a way to reduce exposure to these substances by seeking out the right domestic products, building materials and practices, and even choosing the best regions of the world to live in.

The ubiquity and irreplaceable nature of some of these harmful substances is what makes it so tricky. Take fluoride in toothpaste, for example. Several studies have shown that exposure to fluoride can lead to problematic changes in methylation patterns. First, it can be tricky to find toothpaste that doesn't contain fluoride, and if you do, you also need to be aware of the trade-off, as its teeth and bone mineralization benefits can't be found elsewhere. Take benzene, for example. This is a chemical found just about everywhere: In gasoline and other fuels, paints, lacquer, varnish removers, common solvents, glues, furniture wax, detergents, inks, cleaners, and degreasers. High exposure to benzene has been linked to lymphomas, skin cancers, and leukaemia through the methylation of specific genes. A study on petrol station workers and traffic attendants showed that these groups both experienced heavy methylation of these gene groups and were more at risk of developing these health problems. Even if we don't work these harmful jobs, or in industrial occupations, we are still exposed to these chemicals through basic interaction with the human world. It's simply unavoidable. Some may immediately consider moving to a more remote place to escape environmental pollution, but even this won't do you much good. In fact, some studies on the methylation levels of Inuit peoples in Greenland have actually shown that this population has some of the highest exposure to harmful chemicals.[11] As a result of the Earth's water, wind, and weather systems, pollution in lower latitudes travels up, adding toxins in the North Pole. People who have barely used and benefited from the products containing these chemicals are sometimes those who suffer the worst exposure and health consequences.

Fixing our lives from an epigenetic angle requires scientific research and study, alongside understanding and awareness in people, and widespread availability of viable alternative products. This process of change can be overshadowed by entrenched interests who, for commercial or customary reasons,

---

11 Rusiecki Ja, Baccarelli A, Bollati V, Tarantini L, Moore Le, Bonefeld-Jorgensen Ec. Global DNA hypomethylation is associated with high serum-persistent organic pollutants in Greenlandic Inuit. Environ Health Perspect. 2008;116(11):1547–1552.

want to keep things the way they are, and will lobby against healthier change. That's not to say that widespread public and regulatory action is impossible; there's a list of epigenetically harmful chemicals that have been banned from commercial use: lead in paint, DDT pesticides, asbestos, and dioxin (a herbicide used in Agent Orange). At least we've progressed in some ways. Perhaps the biggest problem is that the list of banned chemicals is longer and more comprehensive in some places than others. Several of the pesticide chemicals in the list above were banned for use in more developed economies but were then actively exported or manufactured for use in developing countries around the world. We may export aid and healthcare, but if we also export banned toxic chemicals, we certainly do more harm than good.

Even within more developed regions, there are wide differences. Europe and the UK have a precautionary approach to chemical pollutants, where a strong burden of proof of human safety is required before a chemical can be used in products. Europe has therefore led the way in controlling pollutants. For instance, several European countries banned lead paint in 1909, whereas the US did not do so until 1978, thus contaminating too many human lives in a 70-year period. The trouble is that in the US, the companies present their own studies and research to the regulatory agency; independent testing is not conducted, meaning the regulator can't test the chemical until it's been proven harmful by the very companies that profit from its use[12], making this a classic case of regulatory capture, and a catch-22 for the health of 330 million Americans.

12https://ensia.com/features/banned-in-europe-safe-in-the-u-s/

That's why there are only nine banned chemicals in the US,[13] all of which were banned between 1978 and 1984. Despite the life-changing advances in human biology, environmental studies, and epigenetics, America has not banned any additional products in nearly 40 years.

Controlling our exposure to chemicals in products and practices is difficult, but nothing is more obligatory and harder to opt out of than the very air we breathe. Particulate Matter (PM) is an output of combustion vehicles and many industrial processes. Regular exposure to this and its correlation to cancer, lung, and heart health have been well-studied. We are now discovering the role this chemical plays in the demethylation of genes, which determine the level of inflammation and oxidative stress in the body. The fewer ribbons, the 'noisier' these genes become, thus causing our levels of cellular inflammation and stress to increase, resulting in overall poorer health.

Serious exposure to air pollution is not just limited to those working in industrial occupations or those living in smog in Asian megacities. The Normative Ageing Study collected over a thousand DNA blood samples from elderly men in the Boston area. An important gene (LINE-1) had lower methylation, which is associated with exposure to black carbon (a common pollutant from traffic). Low methylation in this particular gene has also been determined as a contributing factor for cancers and heart disease. People who live their lives in 'normal' urban areas around the world will suffer the same cellular damage with each breath, slowly but surely disrupting the critical operations of the libraries that keep them living. As urban areas

---

13https://www.businessinsider.com/epa-only-restricts-9-chemicals-2016-2#2-fully-halogenated-chlorofluoroalkanes-2

sprawl, and suburbs overtake the countryside, air pollution is becoming harder and harder to escape. So, the lesson is: Don't panic with each breath. The 'energy of the city' so many of us chase comes at a price, and it's a price paid about 12 times a minute (our average resting breath rate).

Epigenetics

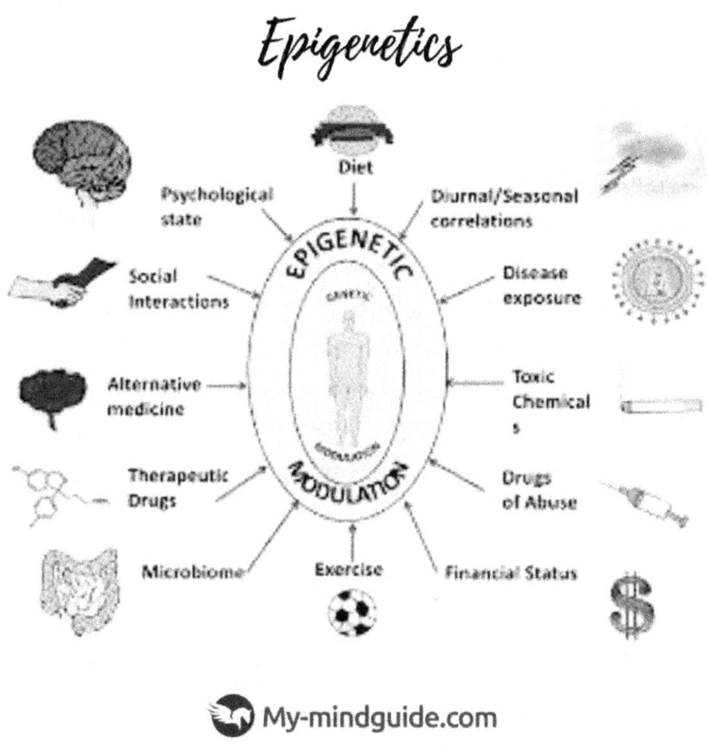

Finally, let's look beyond the evidence on physical environments, and examine how our behavioural and psychological conditions affect our epigenetic landscapes. We'll explore this in more depth with different (less clinical) methods of investigation in the latter part of this book. But here, in the scientific section, it's important to emphasise that we have hard, incontrovertible, and clinical evidence for behaviours and psychological stress physically affecting our bodies through the engines of epigenetics.

People with a history of abuse and stress in childhood have been found to have extreme levels of methylation in the glucocorticoid receptor gene in the hippocampus.[14] Let's unpack those scientific terms. The hippocampus is the area of the brain where we store and process long-term memories, whilst glucocorticoids are vital for maintaining a resting, healthy state, controlling our stress response. So, suicidal victims of childhood abuse have far too many ribbons on genes that help us achieve a calm and restful state away from stress. Importantly, the methylation states of these poor individuals were controlled against suicidal people who didn't experience childhood abuse, and other people who didn't have either problem. On the other note, we've also observed that positive experiences of maternal care lead to less methylation of the same gene, allowing us to better maintain restful states and deal with stress.

These are stressors and traumas that are usually outside of our control. Factors more in our control, such as work hours, are something research has also shed light on. In fact, studies have demonstrated how working at night can negatively affect our epigenetics. Our internal circadian rhythms can become misaligned with the external light-dark cycle of the day, and this misalignment can start to echo into our epigenome. Night shift workers were shown to have altered methylation in genes

---

14Mcgowan Po, Sasaki A, D'alessio Ac, et al. Epigenetic regulation of the glucocorticoid receptor in human brain associates with childhood abuse. Nat Neurosci. 2009;12(3):342–348.

controlling general inflammation.[15] When we choose to be awake—if we have the choice—it affects our epigenome and our long-term health. This explains why our parents always told us to go to bed on time.

So, in this chapter we've explored the major parts of the current scientific boundary of knowledge over how our diet, habits, environment, and psychology affect our epigenome. What's so exciting is that if this chapter was re-written or revised in just five years' time, we'd likely be discussing new determinants and dynamics for the expression of our genes. The boundary of knowledge in this field is shifting day-by-day—so vast and significant is this territory for humans, and so early we are in our quest to map it. Only in the 21st century have we had access to the necessary technology to explore the expression of our DNA on a cellular level, but we've been ruminating on the outcomes of DNA expression for millennia—that is, the outcomes of our lives. We've been building philosophies and systems of thought to try to capture the mechanisms that we can now comprehend in greater detail.

The great minds, the differing perspectives, and the many lifetimes that went into these epigenetic beliefs means they still have value for us today. Exploring this ancient wisdom will lead us down new routes of scientific knowledge—just look at how some of the top epigenetic foods neatly overlap with Eastern systems of medicine. Diet is one thing for science to cover, but behaviour and life decisions are so complex and so difficult to deem scientifically objective, that these ancient philosophies for living a good life will hold merit long into our scientific

---

15 Bollati V, Baccarelli A, Sartori S, et al. Epigenetic effects of shiftwork on blood DNA methylation. Chronobiol Int. 2010;27(5):1093–1104.

future. They enable us to explore how to live, how to work, and even how to conduct research. And so, it's gladdening that, for the most part, our research into epigenetics is led by good intentions for general human health—at least until the machinations of the darker elements of capitalism seek to amplify some parts of the findings, and tirelessly suppress others.

As a species, we do not suffer from a lack of knowledge; we suffer from our own selfishness. Companies use techniques and resources, which we know pollute the environment, not accounting for the damage they do to others. Richer countries know enough to ban chemicals and practices within their own borders, but are happy to profit by exporting them to poorer nations. The people of our time use products, eat foods, and live in a way that steals from the world our children will inherit. We know enough, but we do not yet love enough to act in accordance to these concepts. The following part of this book focuses as much on the latter as the former.

Part Three

The Ancient Understanding of Epigenetics - Other Tools

Epigenetics

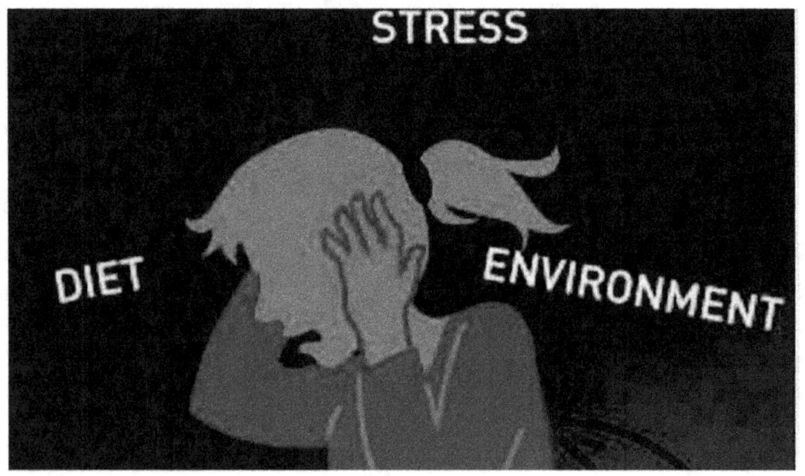

My-mindguide.com

3.1

An Introduction - Why include philosophy and mysticism in a science book?

The journey of understanding we've embarked on thus far has presented us with paths exclusively through the realms of science, both in modern times, and in the relatively recent past. We've come to see how epigenetics lies beyond genetics, and have examined the trail of experiments—both lab-based and accidental in history. All of this has led to our current understanding of the influences and effects of the expression of our genes. We've gone as far as a book like this can go; any deeper or any further, and we'd be getting too complex and too academic for the audience—and possibly even the author!

Modern objective, rational, positivist science is our society's primary tool for investigating and understanding the wonders of life: human, animal, vegetal, or mineral. And so far in this book, we have only used that tool. Everything we've discussed thus far has been accepted by at least a healthy portion of reputable academic researchers. So, as the dominant tool of our society, we have laid the foundations of this book in science. What we venture into now is a more varied, more colourful, more speculative, and possibly more helpful approach to the same subjects we've already discussed.

Science wasn't always strictly dominant as a mode of exploration. Societies had other tools to understand the world with and to live by. And, even in our own times, science may be the primary tool, but it is not the only one.

Now and before, people have used philosophies, religions, myths, stories, music, and visual and performing arts to reflect the external world we live in, and the internal worlds we live through. These fields are also tools for understanding the human experience, for gaining insight into all aspects of life, and for keeping and sharing that received wisdom from generation to generation. But just as with science, these tools of investigation can become corrupted and abused by a select few to manipulate, mollify, terrify, or take value from the general masses. Just as with science, that doesn't mean they can't also be used for great benefit to advance the welfare and lives of humans across the world. And just as with science, we need both the right intentions and the right interpretations of the results for these tools to serve humanity.

In investigating epigenetics—a study of something that has impacted all living things—we'd be missing something if we did not journey through other human realms with these varying tools of investigation. We need to see how humans that were not born into Western society in the 20th and 21st centuries contemplated the same subject, understanding the impact it had on their lives.

Mythmaking, storytelling, and freethinking occur at the boundaries of hard and fast human knowledge. Art is at the edge. What can't yet be understood scientifically is speculated at with other tools of investigation and exploration. Then slowly, as our scientific methods and techniques advance, they start to unravel and penetrate the mysteries that were previously rooted in nothing but myth or religion.

When science advances, myths don't retreat; they just advance to cover even more strange and 'further out' natural phenomena. Take creation myths, for example. Every group of humans generates creation myths, explaining how the world and its inhabitants came to being. Through studying evolution, we've found scientific answers to those questions, and creation myths now serve more creative and reflective— but less explanatory—purposes for many. Science has marched forward and myth has moved on.

We can also look at black holes. Some would say John Mithchell, an English country clergyman, was the first to speculate about these in 1783,[16] whereas Karl Schwarzschild developed the concept in 1916, after Einstein's Theory of Relativity had been published.

That said, Vedic philosophers might disagree with that timeline. One of Shiva's manifestations is Makhala, who represents the dissolution of all things and has the power to subsume time and space into his body. Makhala is usually black in colour, as all colours are absorbed into black, thus representing the absence of light, or—more accurately in the case of a black hole—the absence of light *escaping*. Makhala represents the dissolution of the universe, as after each *kalpa*

---

16 Source: https://www.amnh.org/learn-teach/curriculum-collections/cosmic-horizons
  -book/john-michell black-holes

(or time period of being in light), all is destroyed into the blackness of his body. In this way, Makhala is also the source of being, as all emanates again out of this primordial blackness or *Bindu*. This is conceptually identical to the idea of the singularity in astrophysics,[17] and is well-aligned with the idea of the Big Bang, and the universe expanding—that is, until a great contraction returns us to a massive black hole.

Take these lines of the Rig Veda, whilst keeping the Big Bang in mind:

At first, there was only darkness wrapped in darkness.
All this was only unillumined cosmic water.
That One which came to be, enclosed in nothing,
arose at last, born of the power of heat. (Nasadiya Sukta)

The Rig Veda is thought to have been written around 2000 BC, capturing concepts and Gods that would have been around for millennia. On April 10th, 2019, the Event Horizon Telescope team used eight of the most astrologically powerful telescopes to create a virtual observatory some 12,000 kilometers across to capture a part of space in a galaxy 50 million lightyears away called M87. The resulting image was the first ever photo of a black hole. To a closed-minded scientist or dogmatic religious scholar, these events are unrelated. To those of us with open minds, who can realise we need every tool we possess to understand the complexity and appreciate the beauty of life, they are wonderful human explorations into the same subject.

---

17 https://www.thehindu.com/opinion/columns/what-religious-scriptures-mention-about-black-hole/article61984495.ece

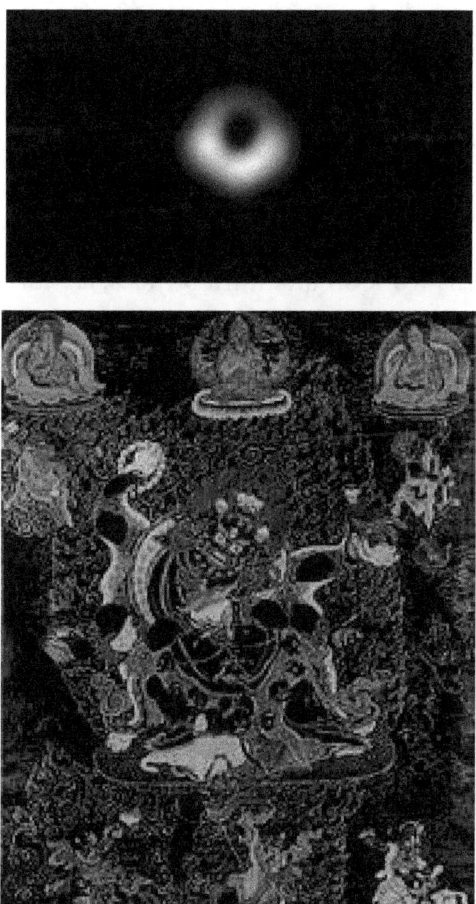

Conveniently distanced from epigenetics, this is just one example where ancient mystical, spiritual, and philosophical contemplation have yielded valuable insight into one of life's mysteries that can stand-up well to modern science, and even enhance our understanding and experience of the concept when used in concert. The deeper we push the boundaries of science, the more we find parallels in ancient thought that half-explained these phenomena millennia ago.

This has been found repeatedly in neuroscience and the question of consciousness, as well as in quantum physics. Werner Heisenberg, the father of quantum physics, told Fritjof Kapra[18] about the time he spent as a guest of Rabindranath Tagore, during which the pair extensively discussed Indian philosophy. Heisenberg explained how these discussions had helped him in developing his work on quantum physics, as *"there was, in fact, a whole culture that subscribed to very similar ideas."*

Niels Bohr, another father of quantum physics, had similar illuminations in China, and with his experiences in Daoism. Indeed, he chose the Ying-Yang symbol as his coat of arms when he was knighted. For human understanding to progress the furthest and the fastest, mythic or mystic philosophy and science should not be perceived to be battling against one another. Rather, they are on the same side—part of the same army—where mystics, artists, and shamans can explore and speculate over a given territory before scientists.

This is how this section seeks to illuminate our emerging understanding of epigenetics. We will see the land through the lens of ancient wisdom rather than detailed clinical trials. The people of the past were as affected by the engines of epigenetics as we are today. They saw its results in their behaviour and lives. What did they think was happening? What systems did they create to explain what was happening in the cell's nuclei (before they knew what a cell was)? How were these systems designed to aid the people in these societies, to act well, and live better?

---

18 The Tao of Physics, Fritjof Capra

3.2

Human Agency - The power of decisions for life

Much of 20th century science has sought purely mechanistic answers when investigating life's big questions. This is because, at first glance, many of life's phenomena are well described by a fairly mechanistic approach. Basic Newtonian mechanics allow us to observe with our eyes, basic telescopes, and microscopes. Now, of course, there are some issues around black holes and subatomic particles, but surely, we can park those aside for the most part.

In its essence, and in very few words, this type of mechanistic thinking sees the world as different collections of bouncing particles. It is a constantly moving ocean of snooker balls, bouncing around off each other to create the phenomena that we observe at our scale of being. And if we can understand how these particles bounce, then we can understand almost any aspect of life: how a ball travels through the air, how salt dissolves in water, and how we digest food into energy.

The most extreme form of this way of thinking then takes aim at us, our brains, and our consciousness. Our brains are cellular matter—collections of bouncing particles—and there are bolts of energy through the synapses of our brain, which lead to actions that translate into what we eat, where we sleep, and who we reproduce with. In this way of seeing the world, we have ascribed total significance to physical matter, and to the atoms that make up things in physical reality. There is no room for any other force, energy, or agency.

This is a very reductive way of seeing the world. If we reduce reality to a bouncing collection of particles, then every bounce, every movement, and every reaction is simply the product of what came before it. There is no decision-making involved; life is simply a mechanical reaction to previous bounces. We have no individual will.

Very conveniently, 20th century scientists that ascribed to this mechanistic way of seeing the world have already dealt with the great question of consciousness. Their case is that human brains evolved through natural selection to become large enough to hunt in big groups and to defend the interests of the group as a whole. The humans who had large enough brains for animal communication and cognition—those sophisticated enough to uphold the complexities of a large tribe—fared better in survival, and so, the average human brain size increased. Now, where does consciousness come from? Well, in the mechanistic scientific view, consciousness of self and other is a mere by-product—a side effect—of these large brains. It's kind of like the pollution that a factory of a sufficient size will create. The smoke is not helpful, purposeful, or meaningful in itself; it's just what happens when a factory of that size operates.

So, where does that leave us, our lives, and our experiences?

Well, it means our conscious experiences are meaningless, boiling the universe down to a large collection of bouncing particles, where reactions are predictable and caused by what happened before. It leaves no space for free-will, or any element or energy that would cause a difference or a diversion off the set path that the universe was on, is on, and will be on forever more. Our destiny is predetermined. The course is fixed. The solution of these 20th century scientific materialists is total, and there is no space left for us.

This way of thinking is an extremely dissatisfactory way to describe the complexities and confusions of consciousness. It is also extremely disempowering for the individual. Living with this mechanistic perspective, or even living around people who hold this perspective, is crushing for the human psyche. It is a plague of modern thought and modern being.

Now, what does the outcome of this philosophical debate sound similar to? What other roads lead to a similarly desperate destination? Genetic determinism means that if a certain type of cancer, or a certain heart disease is written into your genes with a certain likelihood, then you will experience those diseases with that same probability. No action of yours can avert this course; your life decisions are therefore reduced to a meaningless nothing. Believing in the mechanistic view of the universe, and believing in the pure dominance of DNA, are similarly disempowering.

So, what can we do to re-empower ourselves? What type of beliefs and which scientific aspects can bring meaning back into our lives when they've been gutted by mechanistic thinking in physics or biology? In both cases, more modern, advanced science, and more ancient philosophy and systems of thought all point to layers beyond the mechanism. (So, our saviour lies in that which is epi-mechanistic.)

With respect to physics and metaphysics, there is quantum theory, the significance of the observer effect, and the idea of the field of consciousness lying above, within, and around the field of physical matter. If consciousness is not solely derived from the physical system, and the physical examinations of neuroscience have yet to find anything to explain consciousness at a physical level, then it can be the layer of agency or creativity that rescues the universe from pure mechanistic thinking.

Similarly, in biology, we've learned of how recently we've discovered that we are not the product of our genes alone. Through epigenetics, we understand how our actions are significant and crucial in deciding our fate. Our choices impact our lives and others, now and in future generations, rippling across the pool of life. We matter.

So, epigenetics is a scientific and philosophical cure for a wicked type of nihilism that eats everything life can offer when mechanistic thinking takes a deep enough root in our ground of being and belief. The power of genetics is not in doubt; genes are exactly that which have enabled life to occur over billions of years. However, epigenetics is that which brings meaning to self-aware beings who enjoy that life.

So, in practical terms, this is a call to arms—a call to actions—rooted in science and philosophy. You are not helpless. Your decisions are material and vital. But now, you know and understand this. Now, you are empowered. Now, it's your responsibility to educate yourself, act accordingly, and maybe enlighten others, too.

So, where can we look to learn, and who can we learn from? Modern science has been covered well; let's look elsewhere for clues.

3.3

Ancient Knowledge - Epigenetic understanding before the microscope.

Hindu philosophers have long described the experience of "being" as a web—jaal. Genes form the threads of the web; the detritus that adheres to it transforms every web into a singular being. An organism's individuality, then, is suspended between genome and epigenome. We call the miracle of this suspension "fate." We call our responses to it "choice." We call one such unique variant of one such organism a "self."[19]

From *The Gene: An Intimate History*, Siddhartha Mukherjee

For quite some time through the 20th century, modern scientific understanding in the form of genetic determinism blinded and biased us from thinking and examining life in an epigenetic way. In essence, we lost time and opportunities to uncover more about that which guides so much of our lives. This reminds us of something: We may have great tools and techniques for scientific examination, but we are always limited by time. And the greatest limit in time in this respect is the human lifetime. When we experiment on generations of mice, we can do so in weeks or months. But when we examine

---

19 Siddhartha Mukherjee, *The Gene: An Intimate History*

generations of humans and the impact of their decisions, diets, habits, and environments on their lives, we do so in years, decades, and centuries, across multiple generations. For many of us, we simply can't wait that long. Knowing what we do about epigenetics, and how it affects us and our descendants, it's our responsibility to make good decisions and engage in actions that will improve our epigenome.

If our time to act is now, but more data and knowledge is out there in the future, what is left for us in the here and now?

Well, we can let educated guesses rooted in partial knowledge we have now guide the way we act, hoping our estimations fall on the right side of future discoveries. But if we leave ourselves at this juncture, we are being both ignorant and arrogant, disregarding the rest of the iceberg of data because it is not presented to us in peer-reviewed, modern, scientific research papers. The deep well of data that we are ignoring is in our past—all of the lives lived in past centuries, where countless generations came and went, countless habits and behaviours were experimented with, encouraged, let go, or censored. And all the while, there were minds as intelligent, neurologically powerful, and emotionally sensitive as ours to observe, analyse, and record the outcome of their findings across countless types of media. We must remain open-minded, rational, creative, objective, and lucid in our approach to interpreting this fantastic resource of the human past.

Of course, there are major limitations when studying the past in this manner, the first of which is a lack of evidence and information. We must be more holistic with our information sources, insofar as our willingness to use more anecdotal, religious, pictorial, architectural, and other cultural data to establish accurate ideas of the diets, decisions, and behaviours that formed the lifestyles of the past. We have some solid archival and archaeological data to draw on, of course, but we need to use supporting pieces to get to useful places for our purposes.

Since we have enough evidence to do so, we will draw on evidence from the great Indian, Chinese, Egyptian, Greek, Roman, and Islamic civilisations. Where possible, we will also include practices and lifestyle recommendations from other shamanistic traditions around the world. In this way, we can widen the scope of our discussion and consideration on what we would call positive epigenetic practices, observing how these approaches and systems relate to our more recent learnings.

We will leave it to the next section to delve into some specific practices and aspects of life in ancient times that relate to some similar areas that we previously discussed. But first, we need to see the bigger picture. How did ancient societies create wider behavioural and philosophical systems that supported epigenetic living? Put more simply, in times gone by, what was deemed *a good life?*

One of my biggest breakthrough moments was in realising the link between the concept of karma and epigenetics. Here's an excerpt on karma from the Upanishads to start us off:

Now as a man is like this or like that,
according as he acts and according as he behaves, so will he be;
a man of good acts will become good, a man of bad acts, bad;
he becomes pure by pure deeds, bad by bad deeds;

And here they say that a person consists of desires,
and as is his desire, so is his will;
and as is his will, so is his deed;
and whatever deed he does, that he will reap.

— Brihadaranyaka Upanishad, 7th century BCE

Karma is a Sanskrit word meaning 'action' or 'deed'. It is a core concept throughout the Indian religious systems, including Buddhism, but also in Daoism in China. Originally, this term was used to describe how conscious beings (i.e., us) could determine their destinies through the quality and nature of their actions. In essence, karma means that man is master of his fate. When we say, "Our karma," we are referring to the sum of our actions and decisions through our lifetime. The evolution of the term has come to mean that our decisions and behaviours—whether good or bad—will impact our future experience in life accordingly.

Can you see the glittering link to epigenetics here? Karma and epigenetics both hold the same opportunity and danger: Decisions and experiences in your past can imprint themselves in your psyche or on your genes, and can affect your future. Bad decisions and poor habits will echo and cause problems later on. If we adopt a harmful diet, live in toxic environments, experience trauma, or inflict it on others (and therefore ourselves, as well), we are likely to experience the negative ramifications. But there is a positive opportunity there as well. We can clean ourselves and our genes through good action. We have the power to improve our condition. The sages put it best when they said, "*We will reap what we sow.*"

Now, let's go a level deeper. You may already understand how karma is linked to the idea of rebirth, and that there is a well-worn concept of ancestral karma, which is the sum actions of your parents and their parents beyond that. Sound familiar? This notion echoes the core concept of epigenetic inheritance. We inherit our parents' karma or epigenome, and we offer down our own karma and epigenome to our children. It is said that in Kundalini yoga, one soul's healing can liberate seven generations back, and seven generations forward. This also aligns with epigenetics, as research is steadily pushing back the number of generations that can leave an epigenetic trace on our lives, let alone the behavioural and cultural aspects that can clearly be passed down many generations. By fixing these problems in our lifetimes, we may be liberating our children and their children—so to speak—from the genetic and behavioural predispositions that can be passed down through family.

Ancient Indian sages did not have the precise scientific equipment or method to understand this mechanism on a cellular basis. However, they *did* have the wisdom, perspective, and clarity of thought to recognise the outcomes of the mechanism over the course of people's lives and within families. They didn't have to understand methylation or histones; they saw how people's diets, environments, and relationships led to certain outcomes, allowing them to connect the dots into a cogent unified system. If geneticists had paid more attention to karma, we may well have been a few years further ahead in our current lines of research.

Now, India was not necessarily alone in recognising aspects of epigenetics within its spiritual or religious systems; other spiritual traditions held similar concepts. For instance, there's the Christian concept of sin, and *ithm* in Islam, which refers to the belief that God will punish you for your bad deeds in this life and/or the next. Engaging in violence and eating too much of the wrong foods were considered sinful, as was drinking excess alcohol, and living a sedentary lifestyle. So, there were other complete religious systems that echoed tenants of epigenetic principles, but none of these mirrored concepts within epigenetics so directly as karmic law.

So, sin, *ithm*, and even karma were systems for transmitting accumulated wisdom over how best to live. But they were also clearly systems of population control. They gave spiritual and earthly leaders power over people's behaviour. When the punishment for rebellious or disobedient behaviour fell onto your immortal soul, the peasants were more likely to stay in-line. So, as with all religious topics, we need to view these holy laws and mechanisms that lie somewhere on a spectrum between being methods designed by leaders to transmit useful information, and tools for a falsely enlightened few to control the masses by using hell as a stick and heaven as a carrot. This is one aspect of using philosophy and other tools on the hunt for ancient epigenetic understanding. Science, at least, tries to be objective, whereas religion is much less so, meaning we need to be more critical and careful of its true intent.

3.4

—

Self-help of the Ancients - past spiritual practices to wipe the slate clean.

We've addressed why we've included ancient systems of thought in a book on science, why mechanistic and materialist thinking put us in a dark hole, and then how epigenetics can dig us out of it. Finally, we've started to address how the people of the past developed comprehensive systems for how to live, giving general principles to navigate the dangers and opportunities presented by human agency.

But enough preaching—what about practice?

We'll now look at some of the specific behaviours that ancient people engaged in to stay healthy and happy, what the shamans, sages, witchdoctors, wisdomkeepers, priests, and princes prescribed to their people, and how these practices compare to modern ideas and research. These are not strictly epigenetic practices. Instead, these are recommended—and sometimes commanded—practices that were intended for general physical and spiritual wellbeing.

Let's begin with our living environment and personal hygiene. We tend to think of the people of the past as having far worse personal hygiene habits: bathing less often, using less effective sewage systems (if any at all), and living more dirtily in general. Now, in many cases, you'd be right to think this, especially in Europe, where bathing was far less common. However, there is also plenty of evidence of spiritual or religious systems around the world instituting sound personal hygiene habits for their adherents.

For God loves those who turn to Him constantly and He loves those who keep themselves pure and clean. – Quran (2:222].

Cleanliness is half of faith. – Hadith (Prophet Muhammad)

The Islamic religion institutes that followers must wash their hands, feet, and face five times a day before each set of prayers, also referred to as *wudu*. There is also a deeper, full body bath known as *ghusl* that is performed less frequently, such as after intercourse. As such, many Islamic societies constructed public bath houses and washing fountains, many of which are still in use today, such as the *hammams* of Turkey.

Ancient Jews, and some early Christians, also adhered to detailed ritual washing and purification of the body, as recorded in the Old Testament book of Leviticus. It was actually the rebel Jesus who de-emphasised obsessive strictness to these rules, at the expense of love and good human conduct. Perhaps, this was why Christian Europe was one of the dirtiest places in human history. That said, Jesus and his herald/warm-up act, John, were instrumental in spreading the practice of a full-body bath at least once in your life, also known as baptism.

Back in the East, ritual washing and purification were also well-structured into Vedic life, where a caste often defined personal hygiene. In Japan, there are *harae* and *misogi*, which are purification rituals with water in the Shinto tradition. We have another culture now resplendent with ancient and modern spas to rival Turkish hammams: Japanese Onsen.

There is also the Sanskrit concept of *saucha*, which is related to both spiritual and physical purity and cleanliness. *Saucha* implies that one must be careful of the environment, people, and energy they expose themselves to. A whole range of yogic practices were designed and could be performed to cleanse people of impurities—both spiritual and physical—so they could live a healthier and better life.

These concepts don't only refer to the cleanliness of mind and body, but also of house and home. In China, there is the concept of *feng shui*, which constitutes the harmonious re-arranging of a home to reflect and generate harmony within oneself. In Persia, there was the festival of *Nowruz*, celebrated on the Spring equinox, in part by literally shaking the house, or diving into Spring cleaning. We could go on and on with different concepts and practices from societies around the world, where religious or spiritual practices focused and celebrated personal and environmental cleanliness.

It's important to note that many of these concepts of purification draw little distinction between bodily or environmental cleanliness, and that of spiritual, mental, or emotional purity. One was often linked to the other and cleansing one side of this equation was usually thought to help cleanse the other side, as well. This is quite telling. In modern times, we tend to separate wellness and cleanliness.

In times gone by, they were deemed to be far more linked and interdependent, where ritual cleansing had one foot in the physical realm and another in the spiritual. We can learn from this in how orderliness of environment, cleanliness of body, clarity of thought, and purity of heart all run on the same spectrum of wellness. This is backed by what we are finding in modern life studies, which posit that our behaviour and wellness are far more linked than had previously been suggested. We become more emotionally depressed in dirty places, and we know that prolonged exposure to damp and mould can cause epigenetic alterations and bodily disease. This interlinking of different aspects of life is intrinsic to many ancient religious or spiritual practices.

Over the aeons that varying forms of spirituality and religion have been around for, they have had some pretty consistent objectives: peace, joy, serenity, blessings of health, and prosperity. Many world religions also share very similar methods: prayer, mantras, meditation, ritual movement, and chanting or singing. The fact that so many religious groups shared such similar traditions across such vast eras and geographies is likely to suggest that there's some value in them. So many people were unlikely to invest so much time in activities that had little or no practical or spiritual benefits. They must have been able to achieve some of their objectives through these contemplative and affirmative actions.

Let's examine meditation first. Defining meditation is a thankless task—a little like trying to define art. But for the purposes of this discussion, we'll say that meditation constitutes a technique for focusing the mind on an object, thought, or activity to achieve a mentally clear and calm state of being.

This definition does not limit us to Eastern religions (forms of Buddhism or Hinduism) that many in our modern society typically associate with meditation. We can find relevant meditation techniques in almost every religious or spiritual group across the world. Many of the prophets of Judaism are described in meditation in the Torah. Early Greek Christians describe spiritual exercises involving concentration, that extends into medieval monks, as well. *Tafakkur* or *tadabbur* are Sufi techniques for sitting down and reflecting upon the universe and our place within it. They are perceived to be necessary to evolve cognitively and emotionally (i.e., to think more clearly and to be more joyful and loving). We haven't the time nor the words to fully describe the countless other silent, seated, contemplative practices with these aims that are strung out across the world.

We can all recognise how a busy, frantic, and splintered mind leads to overthinking and stress in both the mind and the body. We've already dealt with some of the impacts of stress and trauma in epigenetics, in how trauma in one generation can be passed into another through the epigenome to affect susceptibility to mental and physical diseases. In this way, these meditative practices that shift the mind's attention to a still, often external point of focus are methods for reducing that same toxic stress during the meditation itself, but also leading us to sustained psychological states where we generate less stress, thus making us more resilient to potential stressors in the future. When we are more aware of our mind's movement and focus, we are more masterful of it; we can use it as a wonderful tool, rather than it make a fractured tool of us.

Sages over the ages have recognised that our bodies long for calm and stress-free stages, and so, they designed meditative techniques for our benefit—epigenetic or otherwise—stretching to the present day. In 1979, John Kabat-Zinn, an American student and practitioner of Zen Buddhism, founded the Stress Reduction Clinic at the University of Massachusetts Medical School. He soon renamed the program Mindfulness-Based Stress Reduction (MBSR). He removed any Buddhist references from the course, fully secularising it for a modern Western audience. Lo and behold, the modern practice of mindfulness was born, again aimed at the same objectives as before, but packaged in a way best suited for its intended audience. Its goal was self-awareness.

With awareness comes agency, or the ability to make conscious decisions independent of fleeting desires and whims. Like the decision not to have that cigarette, to go for a walk in nature rather than walking to the pub, to choose the dark fruit smoothie over the chocolate milkshake, or to work out rather than watch Netflix. In having agency and will—2 attributes that result from disciplined meditation—we can make better epigenetic choices. We can consciously build our lifestyle for the good of ourselves and our families. In honing these attributes, we are cutting the keys to a better life.

Now, let's discuss mantra and prayer. Speaking or chanting special phrases in repetition is another hallmark of world religious traditions. In the East, mantras are sacred phrases that can call out or describe aspects of the divine that the person wishes to emulate or bring into their lives.

Let's dive right into a specific example of the world's most famous mantras:

Om Mane Padme Hum

The Dalai Lama has said that this mantra has the power to *"transform your impure body, speech and mind into the pure body, speech and mind of a Buddha."* It roughly translates to, "Praise to the jewel in the lotus." But as with many prayers and mantras, it holds a vast amount of meaning.

Let's break it down syllable by syllable:
Om - the primordial sound of all creation
Ma - dissolving fleeting desire and worldly attachment
Ne - patience and care for ourselves and others
Pad - witnessing without prejudice or judgement
Me - letting go of possessions and focusing on what is important
Hum - the unshakeable and unmovable floor of being

The literal translation of the phrase as a whole is part of the meaning, referring to the spark of life that resides within the heart, that which illuminates us. But each syllable is packed with its own deeper meaning, rich for contemplation. People who use this mantra should not repeat it blindly, and should instead reflect on each of its countless meanings.

There is a physical device linking Eastern mantra with Western prayers, and it is used fairly consistently from Ireland through to Japan: prayer beads. In Asia, the Japanese use *juzu,* other Buddhist and Hindu traditions use *mala,* whilst Catholics use the Rosary. These tend to be beads of some form, or knots, along a length of rope. They are passed through the hand, each bead representing another repetition of the prayer or mantra. In Catholicism, there is a common structure to the Rosary prayer:

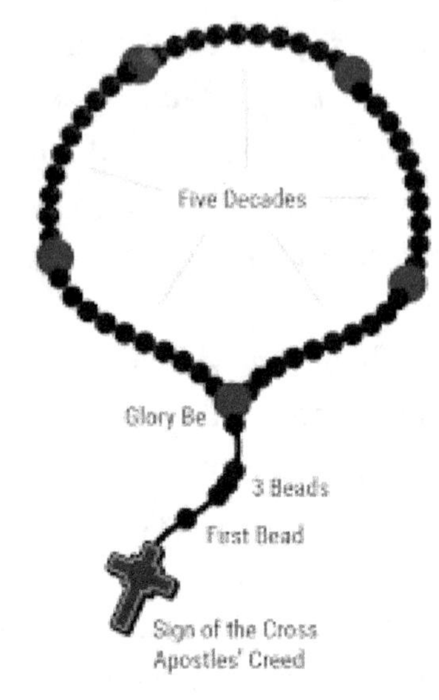

THE PRAYERS OF THE ROSARY

1. The Sign of the Cross - on starting on the crucifix - Blessing oneself and others.

2. The Apostles' Creed - on holding crucifix in the hand) - stating the core beliefs.

3. The Lord's Prayer - at the first large bead - affirming the power and righteousness of God.

4. The Hail Mary - on each of the next three beads - echoing the virtues that Mary demonstrated.

5. The Glory Be - the space before the next large bead - for the glory of God.

This rotation of repetitive prayers using a physical device is, once more, a way of reinforcing the core powers and tenets of Catholic faith. You are blessing yourself, stating what you believe in, stating the total power of your God, reminding yourself of earthly virtues, asking for holy favour, and expressing gratefulness for life itself. These are powerful statements, and repeating them tens or hundreds of times a day will leave a strong and protective mark on your psyche. Through them, you can come to believe in your own righteousness, in the power of the God that you follow, and in how you must behave in this life to achieve the best outcomes.

Although Muslims use prayer beads, or *masbaha,* they also developed other ways to both worship consistently and imprint important concepts onto their psyches. They have the famous call to prayer, *adan,* echoing five times a day from the minarets, *muezzin,* of mosques. This is a community-wide instruction to come and offer prayer, and to collectively reinforce the tenets of Islam and faith in Allah. Here are some approximate translations of excerpts of the daily prayer, *salah,* in Islam:

"Allah is Eternal and Absolute. He begets not, nor was He begotten. And there is none co-equal unto Him."

"Allah hears those who praise Him. O my Lord! Forgive me"

"Peace and Allah's Mercy and Blessings be on you, O Prophet! Peace be on us and on the pious slaves of Allah."

"O Allah, help me to remember You, and thank You, and help me towards the best ways of worshipping You."

Here, again, we have a very similar set of mantras/prayers as in the Christian faith with different framing, in different languages, but after the exact same things.

There are also countless mantras from other less widespread traditions that are targeted towards specific ends. Take the Ho'oponopono of native Hawaianns. It means 'to make things right'. It is a prayer and a Hawaiian practice specifically designed towards forgiveness.

The mantra has four phrases, shortened and translated to:

I am sorry
Forgive me
Thank you
I love you

This phrasing has been used in peace-making, or in resolving trauma, either from the aggressor's perspective, or the victim's. In resolving trauma, it is less important to find the specific faults and details of past transgressions, and more important to dissolve and let go of any remnants of stress that remain in our psyche or within our being. The Ho'oponopono is an ancient method of wiping the slate, of mentally priming to clean past problems, not dissimilar to repenting sins within Christianity. That wiping of the slate is a concept linked to cleaning our epigenome, in taking action and making changes to sever the correlation between a negative past and our incoming future.

There are also several secular hand-me-downs from these traditions of prayer and mantra. In California in the 1970s, two American students at UC Santa Cruz drew together work and teachings from Fritz Perls, a Gestalt therapist, Virginia Satir, a family therapist, and Dr. Milton Erickson, a hypnotherapist. From this eclectic mix of modern healers, they termed the phrase and built the techniques of Neuro-Linguistic

Programming (NLP). NLP is, in essence, a collection of phrases and affirmations to support and develop in various areas of life—be that in family relationships, professional life, personal skills, emotions and confidence, and cognitive abilities. These affirmations and exercises are repeated as with mantra, to imprint positive and attractive thoughts on the brain, and to try to rewire common brain patterns into more productive or positive habits. Of course, it has received its fair share of criticism from conventional medicine, and is classed as an alternative therapy, perhaps to be used in conjunction with other healing methods. But its relationship to traditions of mantra and prayer is extremely close. It is devoid of the mention of God or most other metaphysics, but it taps into the same mechanism.

Another interesting link lies between shamanic drums and brain frequencies. Drums have been used in religious ceremonies worldwide for millennia. They have given rhythm to chants around the fire from the dawn of human history. Men and women often depend on the beat of the drum to achieve altered states of consciousness, where they seek to work in different realms and with different spirits to achieve outcomes in the material world. A related technique was developed in the 1940s and 1960s by Jose Silva, a radio technician living in Laredo, Texas. Silva combined his knowledge of radio frequency with what was coming out of the emergent field of neuroscience, and his personal study of Rosicrucianism, alchemy, and other esoteric groups. He built a technique based on sound waves, mantras, and hypnosis to alter his students' brain states. His technique could slow the cycles of people's brains through the common frequency bands of mental activity. Modern neuroscience is now recognising how the varying states of brain frequency serve respective purposes within our life, some of which are related to calm homeostasis, or memory and learning, or indeed deep healing of the body. Silva was harnessing this and offering positive programming or mantra recitation at suitable moments to affect psychological states. After decades of practice, experienced meditators have been found to skilfully switch between brain states. Silva was using sound frequencies to grant relative novices the same abilities. It's fascinating to now see how shamans' drumbeats can echo these frequencies throughout different parts of their own ceremonies. Humans have been trying to harness the power of the mind and its relation to frequency to influence the body, all while using the technologies that were available in their respective times.

So, here we have yet another example of people from our day and age building on life-improvement techniques from the past, but harnessing them to the technological advances of today. Be it in the hum of a mantra or a modern affirmation, in the clicks of Silva's machines, or from the beats of a shaman's drums, we can hear the desire to better our way of being. These are ways of rewriting patterns of thought and behaviour, reinforcing that which we aspire to be, and dropping what we want to leave behind. They are ways of making change happen—change that starts in the mind, echoes throughout the body, and ends on the epigenome.

We've delved into how we perceive and relate to ourselves, but what about how we relate and treat others? How do the quality of our relationships impact our epigenome, and what provisions did past peoples put in place to form and celebrate the bonds that protect and heal us?

In section 2.4, we examined the potential adverse epigenetic impact of trauma and extreme stress, but we didn't cover loneliness and poor community relationships. Research is now uncovering the dynamics that interplay between genetics and epigenetics regarding loneliness.[20] On the one hand, scientists have found specific genes that make people more sensitive to feeling alone through neurological factors, and these same drivers can also cause people to become more isolated. On the other hand, scientists are also uncovering an epigenetic angle, where social isolation and a lack of community relationships can—through your epigenome—exacerbate cognitive decline, raise stress levels, and put you at a higher risk of developing cancer. These findings were discovered in a study on rats that had been given low levels of maternal care, in turn demonstrating lower levels of methylation.[21]

The importance of community and familial relationships was well understood and deeply embedded in pre-industrial communities around the world. They may not have explicitly understood some of the biological processes of loneliness, but in their empathy and intuition, the emphasis placed on maintaining the full spectrum of community relationships dwarfs our typical modern ways. There is the universal, pre-modern adage of having 'respect for the elders', which appears in almost all religious law. Elderly people are also of those most prone to loneliness, since their friends and 'upstream' family members are more likely to have already passed. What is left is their 'downstream' family, and in traditional societies, elderly people were cared for more closely out of both culture

______

20 https://www.apa.org/science/about/psa/2017/09/loneliness-sick
21 https://www.researchgate.net/publication/8055512_Maternal_Programming_of_Individual_Differences_in_Defensive_Responses_in_the_Rat

and necessity. Tribes were more closely knit and reliant on one another than local modern communities, and so, harmonious relationships mattered that much more. Elderly people were also depositories for wisdom because far fewer people had access to written resources at the time, and so, older people were afforded more respect for their knowledge and experience, as there were often no other ways to access the past but through living memory.

In showing care and respect across generations, we are not just acting in the benefit of our family; we are also putting in place safeguards on loneliness, and all its ill-effects on health. We are retaining insight from one generation to another, and we are protecting our culture, which, in itself, has epigenetic impacts around trauma and identity. When a people lose elements of their native culture—be it organic, through modernisation and globalisation, or more violent, through oppression or cultural genocide—the resulting trauma in lacking an identity and belief system to explain the world can be destabilising for people and their wellbeing. You can take a trail of tears through the stories of Indigenous peoples around the world and find countless examples where a people's culture was torn from them, disbanding their life. When the epigenetic research is eventually done, I suspect there will be strong traces of these events and traumatic processes on people's epigenomes, both from their original loss, and the toxins that these people are then exposed to in modern life.

Take the plight of Native Americans, for instance, many of whom experienced the original 'trail of tears' in being moved off the fertile forests of the American South-East, forced to march across the country to Indian reservations on the arid plains and deserts of the Midwest. Their children were forced into re-education schools, where any native culture was strictly prohibited, whilst distilled alcohol (and then opiates) became the effective currency on these reservations. Even today, very few public services for health or education are available on the reservations, and many people's primary food sources are gas station markets selling cheap, ultra-processed foods. This combined psychological and physiological damage travels beyond cultural genocide, and can be classed as a (epi)genetic genocide. Just as we found traces of the Holocaust on the epigenome of survivors' children, so too will we find these effects elsewhere around the world, within the human wreckage left in the wake of globalisation.

Now, before we can progress to our next domain of learning from ancient practices—our diet—we will first focus on what these people *didn't* eat—the ancient and near-universal practice of fasting.

We have evidence of fasting rituals in Ancient Greece, Pre-Columbian Peru, and amongst Native American cultures. In Ancient Egypt, there was evidence of spiritual men fasting in the desert 'to dry out' and then replenish their bodies. In Native America, young tribe members fasted in the wilderness for four full days on vision quests to connect with the land's spirits. There is lent in Christianity, and perhaps most famously, Ramadan in Islam. In both faiths, the traditional fast revolves around only eating when the sun has set. The traditional Black Lenten Fast in Christianity involves one meal at sundown, whilst Ramadan involves one meal at sundown, *iftar*, and one meal before dawn, *suhoor*. For the rest of the day, all food is avoided; alcohol, meat, and dairy are also variously prohibited.

Ramadan lasts for 30 days a year, whereas Lent lasts for 40. These are society-wide, institutionalised, annual practices within these traditions for the purposes of health, reminding us of the value of food and of the importance of helping those less fortunate.

However, up until very recently, in the modern secular West, fasting as a practice for wellbeing was almost unheard of. Many thought you were mad and surely going against doctor's orders if you weren't consuming three meals a day.

But as with so many customs, in this chapter and beyond, the very latest science is starting to heartily agree with the ancient practice; fasting can be fantastic for your health. First, in a society with widespread obesity, any method to reduce the calories that we consume will derive immediate health benefits through weight loss. Beyond this, there is fasting's role in allowing our organs and digestive systems to rest and repair themselves. We can now track their improved function after periods of fasting. This includes improved control of blood sugar and insulin response. Fasting has also been proven to reduce inflammation, a key marker of multiple diseases. It has also been shown to be beneficial for the heart and our cholesterol, as well as brain function, and in preventing neurodegenerative disorders. There is the effect of cellular autophagy, whereby the cells in our bodies run out of glucose-based fuel, and instead, our cellular machinery uses the protein junk in our cells as a fuel source. In the long run, this improves the lifetime operation of the cell, helping to prevent cancer. It is also well established that fasting can increase the lifespans of many organisms, from bacteria to mice and other mammals. As usual, definitive human evidence is hard to come by, but all evidence points to the notion that fasting enhances human life.[22] There has also been some limited research on the epigenetic impact of fasting practices, where improved methylation patterns were seen to result from such a practice.[23]

As you may have noticed, these benefits are starting to gain mainstream attention after fasting was picked up out of the sands of time by body-hackers, futurists, and entrepreneurs in Silicon Valley. Fasting is making a comeback in a big way, to prevent illness through a regular lifetime practice, and also as an alternative course to cure early onset cancer. Our predecessors were well aware of these benefits that fasting afforded, as well as other potential 'spiritual superpowers'. But with the industrial day, in its rota of mealtimes and all else, as well as with the effect of steady secularisation, we lost the regular practice of fasting. Only now are we partaking in the incredibly simple but effective decision not to eat, seeing what the wisdom of an empty plate has to offer us.

When it does come to eating, we are also starting to look at the food of our forefathers in a new light. The science of epigenetics is shining this light, as well as the emerging concept of nutrigenomics, dieting for the good of our genome. As we already discussed in earlier chapters, many of the epigenetic ingredients of nutrigenomics show a strong overlap with revered medicinal foods from cultures around the world. Look at cacao, for instance, as used by the Aztecs, Mayans, and other Mesoamerican cultures in ritual and worship. Cacao is

---

22 https://www.ncbi.nlm.nih.gov/pmc/articles/PMC6515465/

23 https://clinicalepigeneticsjournal.biomedcentral.com/articles/10.1186/ s13148-017-0340-8#:~:text=Conclusions,NBW%20but%20not%20LBW%20 subjects.

a rich source that the body uses to regulate DNA methylation, also impacting mRNAs levels of DMNTs.[24] Partly because of new scientific discoveries, and partly because of a renaissance in rituals, we have brought raw cacao back into regular consumption.

Then, there's curcumin or turmeric root, as discussed in the previous chapter. This is known as the 'golden spice' in Ayurveda, both because of its colour and because of its many uses. It is used across the whole of Asia—from Afghanistan through India, to China and beyond—in traditional medicine to treat a range of health conditions, and to ensure continued health. Now, we've found curcumin as an effective antioxidant, as well as having anti-microbial and anti-inflammatory properties.[25] Indeed, the ramping up of interest in turmeric has been fairly extreme with 3000 academic publications focusing on it over the last 25 years. And this is part of a wider trend, where more and more modern doctors are starting to see food as the primary form of medicine, to be used well before interventions with synthetic drugs. A rapid route to research success in nutrigenomics would be to start studying the properties of the primary ingredients in traditional herbal medicine. This has already attributed several powerful, scientifically backed dietary aids to epigenetic function, and it will continue to do so.

Again, this original success doesn't boil down to the precise, microbiological science of ancient cultures, but instead offers close observation over many lifetimes of the effects of nature's

---

24 https://www.ncbi.nlm.nih.gov/pmc/articles/PMC3694105/
25 Sahdeo Prasad and Bharat B. Aggarwal, *Herbal Medicine: Biomolecular and Clinical Aspects.* 2nd edition

botanical riches on human health and illnesses. These insights come from a combination of time, intelligence, and an openness that is not always present in the modern scientific mind. We would do better in this field if we could recognise this wealth of insight that has been passed down through the ages.

Now, we've saved perhaps the most remarkable, most recent, and most dramatic rediscovery of an ancient epigenetic tool for last. This is a spiritual tool that differed slightly across the continents in form but was always used for similar ends in settings that were much alike. It is incredibly ancient, and many modern-day scientists now believe it to be fundamental in advancing human consciousness and building our self-awareness. Despite its integral role in tribal cultures around the world, it was not widely propagated in large monotheistic societies, where religion was at least as focused on controlling the masses as it was in spiritual healing or evolution, thus making this tool somewhat problematic.

Up until very recently, this technology was actively prohibited, tightly controlled, and highly stigmatised, and still is, to some extent. Research into its enormous therapeutic potential has restarted in earnest only in the last decade. Many psychologists, neuroscientists, and pharmacologists have been touting it as something of a silver bullet for the greatest causes of disability in the modern age: depression and anxiety disorders. So, what is it? We are, of course, talking about the ritual and therapeutic use of psychedelics.

A comprehensive examination of the human use of psychedelic plant medicine can't be covered in a single book. It would require more of an encyclopaedia. However, we can provide some highlights of its use around the world, offering pathways for individual exploration afterwards. The first posited semi-deliberate ingestion of psychedelics by humans is thought by many to be the most important, and took place across the African savanna and woodlands around a hundred thousand years ago. There is a problem in human intelligence and awareness, whereby we've had the same neurological hardware—the same brain size and structure—for far longer than we've exhibited signs of advanced consciousness and self-awareness. We are, therefore, left looking for some sort of trigger that activated or altered our brains into the language-speaking, large group-forming, myth-making, art-creating, self-aware individuals we are today. One theory—now increasing in both evidence and supporters—is that wild psychedelic fungi were largely responsible for activating this shift in human consciousness. After steady, often accidental dosing of naturally available psychedelics, we began to develop more complex forms of language and symbols, our eyesight and recognition of colour and form changed, and our emotional complexity and ability to form larger groups was established. This is, in brief, the *stoned ape hypothesis*, giving a glimpse into the potential significance of psychedelics in human history.

Let's move on to more deliberate use of psychedelics within ritual settings around the world. There is a rich tradition of psilocybin use across Mesoamerica. This is where Robert Gordon Wasson, a Vice-President at J.P. Morgan and an amateur mycologist, met María Sabina, a Mazatec curandero and shaman, in 1957. Morgan was the first modern Westerner to take 'magic mushrooms' in a ritual setting. Psilocybin was used to initiate the young into the mysteries of life, but also as a regular medicine for adults to ward off evil spirits and demons. For the shamans of Siberia and the Arctic, psychedelic mushrooms were ritually consumed to enter altered states and resolve problems therein. They were also distributed to tribe members for consumption at certain times of the year, most particular the winter solstice, when the old year died and the new one was born. This was likely an opportunity for people to drop any problems of the past year behind them, and to set new ambitions and intentions for the year ahead. This has now been proven to be the origin of Father Christmas and his reindeer. The psychedelic mushrooms were red in colour with white specks, whilst the shamans that distributed their wisdom and the fungi rode on sleds that were often pulled by reindeer, all whilst wearing shamanic costumes. The consumption of mushrooms brought fresh insight into old problems, and brought gifts of wisdom from the altered state. It's fairly clear to see where the different symbols of our own modern pagan Christmas myth emerged.

Across the Amazon lies the mother of all psychedelics, ayahuasca, which, in its active chemical form, is DMT, combined with monoamine oxidase inhibitors (MAOIs) that prolong the activity of DMT in the body. Rainforest tribes that use ayahuasca, or 'the vine of the dead', record the ways in which it is a sacred technology that was shown to them by the Gods. It is, indeed, remarkable that they were able to find and collect the two plants amongst thousands of jungle species, that when combined and prepared in multiple stages, lose their toxicity, and instead create prolonged and deep altered states in the human brain.

In carefully structured ritual settings, ayahuasca is used to dispel evil spirits, thus restoring health, balance, and serenity to the previously troubled individual. Ayahuasca had a strong impact on every aspect of these people's existence, from their medicinal and metaphysical systems, through to the temple architecture, which reflects the geometric shapes of users' hallucinations of the plant. Much is the same for Peyote or San Pedro, hallucinogenic cacti with mescaline as the active ingredient, used in rituals by Native Americans across the Southern Plains and Mexico for at least 5000 years. The plant medicine is central to the life practices of these people, for it brings them closer to God and heals them.

Moreover, in Ancient Greece and Rome, there were the Eleusinian mysteries and Dionysian cults, where citizens gathered once a year to drink ergot wine. Fascinatingly, initiates were only permitted to attend the ceremony once in their lives, and they had to simply make the most of their one-time access to the Gods. The initiates of both groups form a very illustrious list, including Sophokles, Herodotus, Aristophanes, Plutarch (Eleusinian Mysteries), Alexander the Great, and Spartacus (Cult of Dionysius).

Before we head into the current wave of medical interest in some of these psychedelic plants, it's worth taking a brief tour through the West's stance on them in the second half of the 20th century, and well into the new millennium.

Albert Hoffman discovered LSD in 1943. In 1957, Wasson brought back psilocybin into the Western realm. Ayahuasca and Peyote had much later introductions. Thereafter, the number of clinical trials steadily increased, as mid-century pharmaceutical companies (and militaries) started to realise the power and potential of these substances. Then, there was the Summer of Love in 1967, when LSD and—to a lesser degree—psilocybin enjoyed unregulated and increasingly widespread use across Western youth. However, in 1971, President Nixon initiated the War on Drugs in the US, and equivalent legislation spread through Western Europe shortly after. During this time, propaganda claimed that psychedelics caused AIDS, madness, homosexuality, and instant death. To be drunk in the streets was seen as infinitely safer than taking a tab of acid at home. The War on Drugs was raging, and as with many late 20th century wars, the West had initiated it. This war could have subdued the enemy at great cost to itself, but in the end, it had to beat a quiet retreat, and then attempt to polish that defeat as a strange type of victory.

We can now come to that same quiet retreat, also referred to as the psychedelic renaissance that we in the epicentre of. Had we listened and learned from cultures that kept their ancient wisdom alive and well through their elders, we could be 70 years—or several centuries (depending on perspective)—ahead of where we stand now. But before we get too deep into this, let's examine some of the recent studies on psychedelia.

Unsurprisingly, mental conditions and diseases have been the primary targets of this research because these drugs are primarily active within the brain. This is quite timely, considering that the rates of clinically diagnosed depression and anxiety disorders increased by around 50% globally from 1995-2015, and then tripled in America during the Covid-19 pandemic.[26] Conventional medicine has been using SSRIs, or synthetic opiates, to keep these conditions in check. However, these drugs do little to fix these issues, and simply manage the pain. They are also highly addictive, and their widespread prescription has led to a host of social problems around the

---

26 https://www.apa.org/monitor/2021/11/numbers-depression-anxiety

developed world. LSD, psilocybin, and ketamine have all been involved in clinical trials, demonstrating significant and prolonged impact in fixing these mental diseases after as little as one dose. Moreover, these drugs are not addictive, and have little to no side effects. They tick many of the boxes from a pharmaceutical standpoint, failing in just one: these are well-known, easily reproducible, but crucially unpatentable substances. Any profits made from selling these medicines to people will be marginal, as multiple companies will compete in marketing them.

There's a lot more to cover here on the clinical application of psychedelics, yet this book's focus is on the specific epigenetic angle of these ancient technologies for wellbeing, so that's where we'll head. As well as modulating brain activity and neurotransmission, DMT has also been shown to influence gene expression and epigenetic regulation. DMT activates the sigma 1 receptor (SIGMAR1), which is a gene receptor that also responds to stress, promotes cell survival, protects the brain, and aids neural plasticity. When DMT is combined with a MAOI, as in ayahuasca, it can make the areas of the brain where we store negative memories turn hyperactive, so that we can isolate and retrieve these memories. This is aligned with what test subjects experience, which can be a sort of replaying of negative episodes from their life. The difference is that this time, the SIGMAR1 receptor is firing on all cylinders. SIGMAR1 interacts with the HDACs, who are responsible for taking post-it notes off the scroll spools, or in scientific terms, histone deacetylation. This means that the histones can be more tightly packed together, allowing DNA in the cells of the amygdala (the brain's fear centre) to be remodelled. For this reason, SIGMAR1 is a powerful aid to neuroplasticity. When

SIGMAR1 is fired up, parts of the brain are in a state open to change.[27] So, the memory is replayed, but now, there is an opportunity to disconnect the trauma and fear response from that memory, thus healing it. This also allows for the cellular instructions to be updated not to start a fear response when that synapse is fired, or when that trigger is encountered in real life.

This potential mechanism could make ayahuasca an incredibly effective medicine for targeting and fixing complex and severe cases of PTSD. Due to its epigenetic effects and its modulation of the immune response, medical researchers are also excited to apply it to other conditions where cellular memory and operations have broken down, including cancer, diabetes, autoimmune and neurodegenerative disorders, and substance addictions. But let's not limit ourselves to ayahuasca; we can also take on a drug that has a longer and more well-known history in Western consciousness: LSD.

In recent work on mice, micro doses of LSD were found to "reverse stress-induced retraction of dendritic spines in the prefrontal cortex."[28] This means that after stress or trauma, the connective parts between synapses in a crucial area of the brain for decision-making and personality can become damaged or loosely connected. This makes us less open-minded, and more ruled by fearful habits. We become less social, more depressed, and more sensitive to stress—a common set of symptoms in many people suffering from mental diseases. However, even

---

27   https://www.frontiersin.org/articles/10.3389/fphar.2018.00330/full

28   De Gregorio D, Inserra A, Enns JP, et al. Repeated lysergic acid diethylamide (LSD) reverses stress-induced anxiety-like behaviour, cortical synaptogenesis deficits and serotonergic neurotransmission decline. Neuropsychopharmacology. 2022;47(6):1188-1198.

very small, barely perceptible, doses of LSD were able to reverse this, improving the connective ability of synapses in mice. In a very similar experiment with psilocybin,[29] researchers stated the following: *"We not only saw a 10 percent increase in the number of neuronal connections, but also they were on average about 10 percent larger, so the connections were stronger as well."* Even more importantly, these changes were still around a month after the dose was administered—a very long time for rodents.

For psilocybin and LSD, the important gene and enzyme in action is called mTORC1. This also promotes neuroplasticity, as is involved in creating proteins or cellular machinery. It's like the designer that sends the instructions to make the machine, which in turn creates new neurons. If the designer is encouraged by ingesting LSD and psilocybin, then the effect ripples down the chain, and we can see big changes quickly. Also, from an epigenetics angle, scientists have been able to directly quantify the impact of LSD on the methylation of hundreds of genes, many of which regulate neuronal growth and development. To sum it up, the scientists in the study stated how these substances *"prime the brain for integrating new psychological experiences,"* enabling real change in the brain, the body, and the life, to occur.

Now, much of this research can be mediated by the fact that it is primarily been tested on rodants and other small creatures.

However, there is a slew of therapeutic evidence emerging from human use in clinical settings. What is more—and this is key—is that these are not new medicines. People from

---

29https://www.cell.com/neuron/fulltext/S0896-6273(21)00423-2

around the world have been using these substances to heal for thousands and thousands of years. The medicine men of these cultures have run thousands upon thousands of successful treatments on people with many different problems from a range of backgrounds and ages. The evidence and data are there, just not in conventional form accepted by modern Western medicine. Moreover, pharmaceutical companies are struggling to find the best way to patent and profit from these openly available substances.[30] How these substances are corporatized and released into the medical realm will likely be very telling of the problematic world we live in. Psychedelics are perhaps the starkest example of an epigenetically active technology that has been ignored until only very recently.

The people of the past had luxuries that we in modernity will struggle to enjoy ever again. They had time. Time to watch, study, and reflect without the bombardment of thousands of possible distractions and pieces of information, all accessible without even standing. They had time to experiment, developing slow-burning, lifelong techniques for improving their lives and those of their people. They had less information and could perhaps think more clearly. Also, they shared information in deeper ways than many of us do now with one another. They shared stories between generations, and maintained and innovated complex rituals and ceremonies that we have just the echoes of. Our rituals today are often shorn of the meaning and transformative power behind their symbols .

The world is moving so fast now—so fast that things can be left behind much more easily. At that speed of movement, there

---

30https://harvardlawreview.org/2022/02/patents-on-psychedelics-the-next-legal-battlefront-of-drug-development/

is stress. And when there is stress, there is anxiety. This change can be violent, and because it's violent, it can also be traumatic. Now, more than ever, is the time to focus on and value the techniques and tools that enable our bodies and minds to deal with the rapid, stressful, and sometimes traumatic change we are experiencing.

Change is not easy. Achieving deep, lasting, positive change can be even more difficult. It can sometimes take years—decades even—of meditative, contemplative, or mantra-based practice to achieve states of consciousness that can be reached directly by the consumption of certain psychedelic substances. And if these states of consciousness are places where we can enact epigenetic changes, then psychedelics are a powerful and accessible tool indeed.

But even the most vocal proponent of medicinal psychedelics would not recommend them in isolation. For us to be properly equipped to deal with the trials and tribulations of life on earth right now, we need to use every tool in our inventory. We need to each build a comprehensive set of practices, individually suited to to our lives, while also drawing on the insights of science, and the wisdom of those who came before us. We may consume psychedelics to initiate positive change, but to maintain it, we will need to mix in mantra and affirmation, prayer and meditation, dance and exercise, and care over our diet and environment.

As Gandhi's old adage goes, *"If you want to change the world, then start with yourself."*

And we can change ourselves. We've learned in this book how deeply it is possible to change ourselves, right down to our DNA, both positively and negatively. We've also learned of all the different things that *do* change our DNA, as well as the impact they have on us, whether we like it or not. We have the ability to make life decisions, which in turn will determine those dynamics that write themselves onto our epigenome. After we've consciously reclaimed agency in our lives, we can decide what we eat and drink, whether we exercise and how, where we live, who we spend time with, what we place our attention on, which thoughts we have, and how we feel about them. All of this will determine our epigenome, which will echo through our lives and those of our descendants.

Yes, we can change ourselves, which will change the world. But no man is an island, and we are each and all one cell in the great organism of Planet Earth. In making this change in ourselves and in the world, we will need community. We need others to learn from, and to teach to. We need to find those who are open to themselves and others, accountable to themselves and others, and loving to themselves and others. These are the people who can help us drive positive change, both within our bodies and outside in the world.

If you enjoyed this title and would like to read about other topics that have changed my life, please check out my new books on Amazon or my website: www.my-mindguide.com.

Also, let's stay connected on social media. Please drop a line on Facebook or Instagram, and stay tuned for updates! You're welcome to share your thoughts with me directly, as well: gassner@my-mindguide.com. In return, I'll send you a gorgeous infographic that you can cut out and frame.

Also, please leave a review on Amazon, as this will help me reach an even broader audience. Thank you so much for your time, insight, and undying hunger for knowledge!

I want to say thank you to my colleagues, clients, friends, and family members, who have all contributed to what I am now.

I also want to say thank you to Gabriel Palacios, the king of hypnotherapy and a Swiss bestseller author who taught this old fox new tricks, letting me deep-dive into the mystery of hypnotherapy. I learned so much along the journey that I'm now a certified master-hypnosis and conversation coach myself!

Furthermore, I want to say thank you to the fantastic teachers of SAMYANA/Bali who trained me to become a certified yoga and meditation teacher.

Last but not least, I give a special thanks to my master-teacher, Eckhard Wunderle, who's close to a saint to me. He introduced me to the world of meditation, and let me discover all the wonders it has to offer. I couldn't be prouder about having received my certification as a meditation teacher directly from him at the Institut für Spirituelle Psychologie.

Peace, love, and happiness to all of you—'till next time!

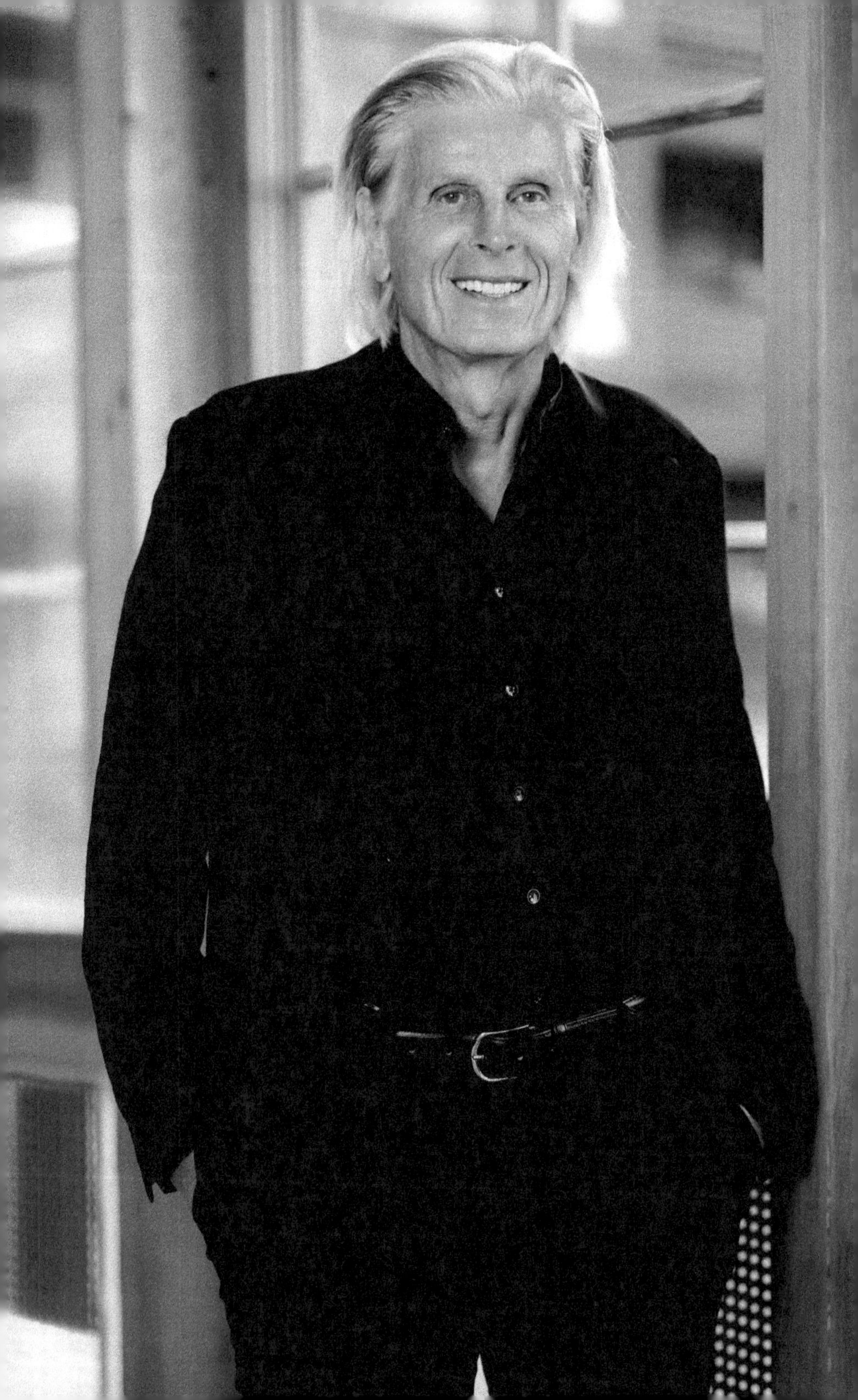

About the Author

Kurt Friedrich Gassner has worn many hats throughout his lifetime, including but not limited to serial entrepreneur, Cceative director, meditation teacher, licensed hypnotherapist, and more recently, self-improvement author. Leveraging his treasure trove of experiences and in-depth knowledge of psychology, he provides his readers with the tools they need to unlock their infinite potential.

As a prolific self-help writer, Gassner has authored the following books: *The Power of Forgiveness, Lie or Die, Soul-Match, A Poisoned Mind?* and *The Power of Poverty.* He has also authored a best-selling children's book in German-speaking countries, and has over 20 books underway.

When it comes to enduring success, Gassner understands that financial prosperity isn't the only aspect one should strive for. He may be a self-made millionaire, but what really transformed his life was mastering his unconscious mind. Perseverance, personal power, self-awareness, and learning from past mistakes have all been key ingredients to bringing his dreams to fruition—and he strives to impart that wisdom onto others through his writing.

During his spare time, Kurt Friedrich Gassner is either travelling across the globe, golfing, biking in the Alps, hiking, or spending quality time with his loved ones. He has been happily married for the last 37 years, and is the father of two successful children. Presently, he resides in Munich, Germany, and Kirchberg, Austria.

https://en.wikipedia.org/wiki/Kurt_Gassner

OTHER BOOKS BY THE AUTHOR

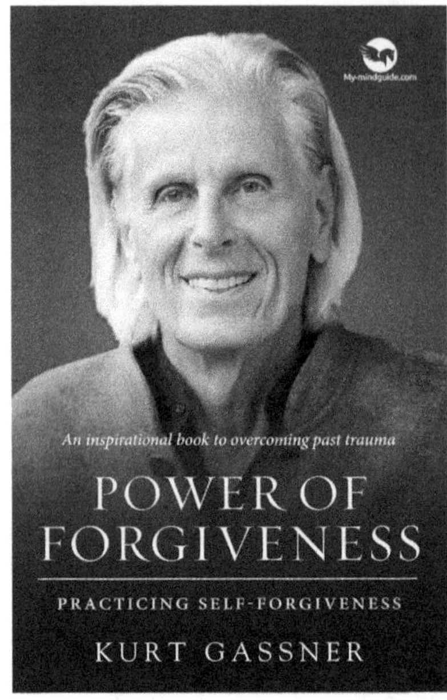

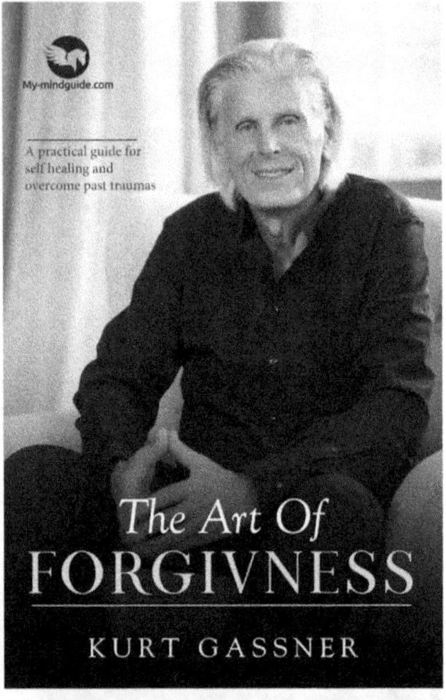

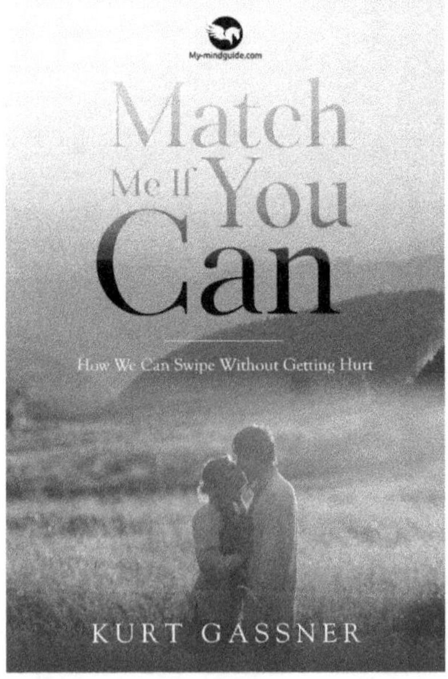

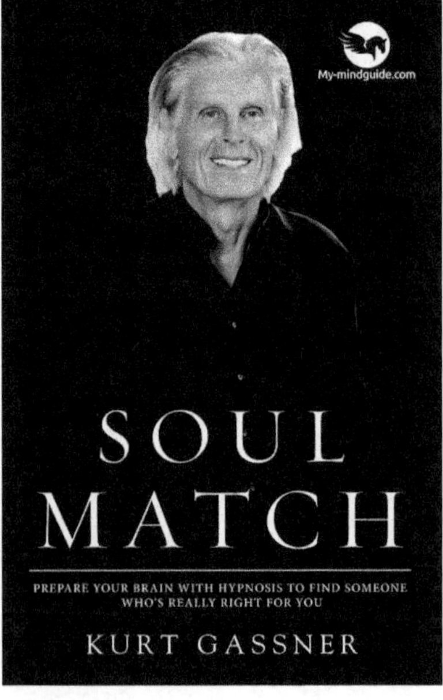

OTHER BOOKS BY THE AUTHOR

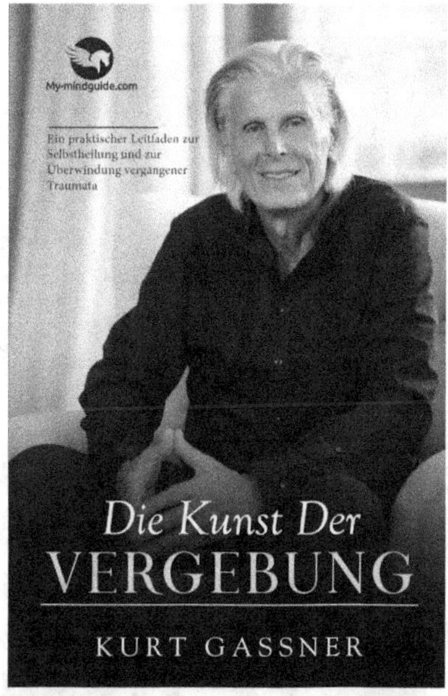

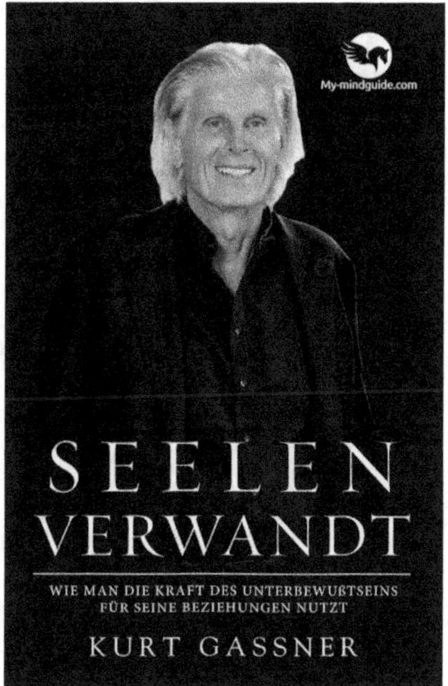

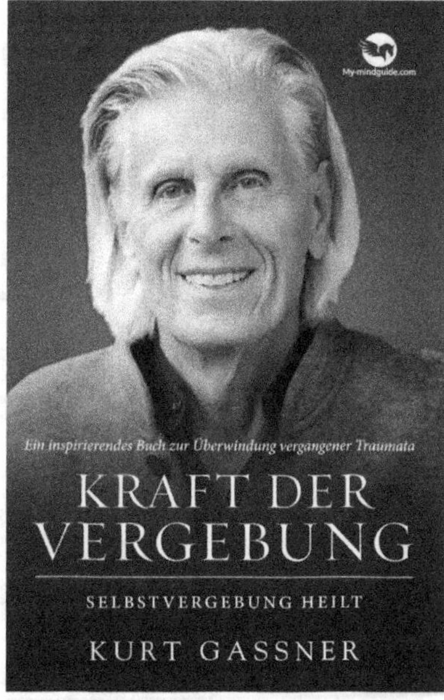

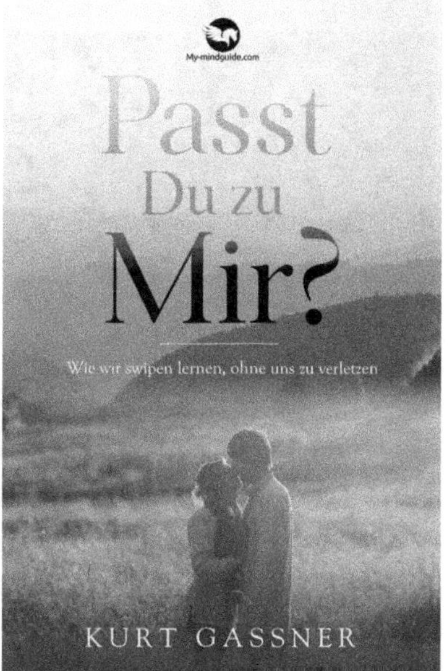

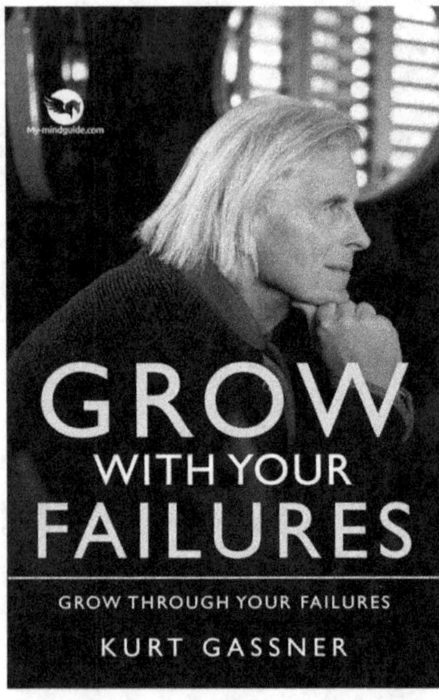

GROW
WITH YOUR
FAILURES
GROW THROUGH YOUR FAILURES
KURT GASSNER

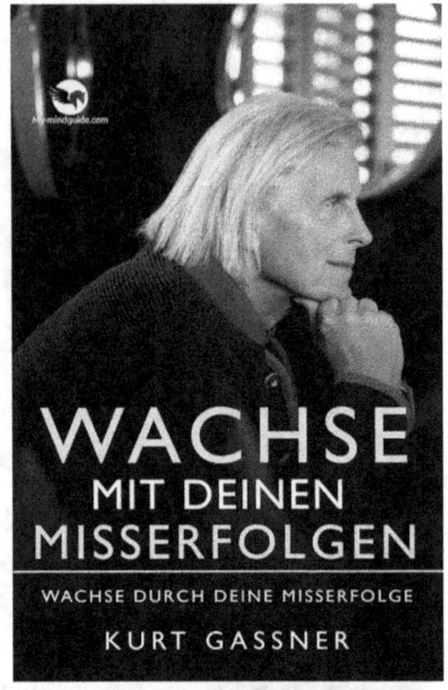

WACHSE
MIT DEINEN
MISSERFOLGEN
WACHSE DURCH DEINE MISSERFOLGE
KURT GASSNER

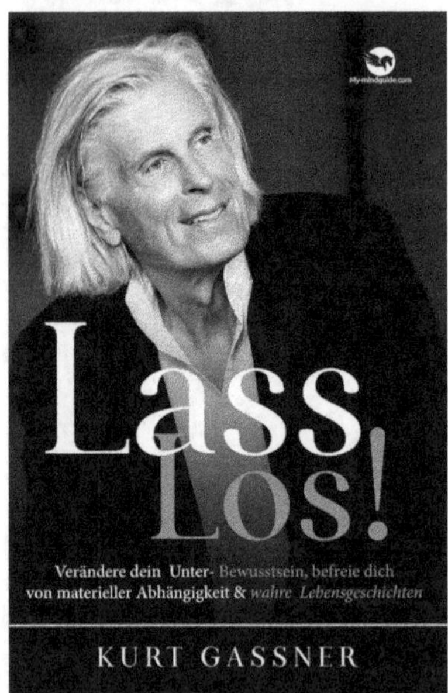

Lass
Los!
Verändere dein Unter- Bewusstsein, befreie dich
von materieller Abhängigkeit & wahre Lebensgeschichten
KURT GASSNER

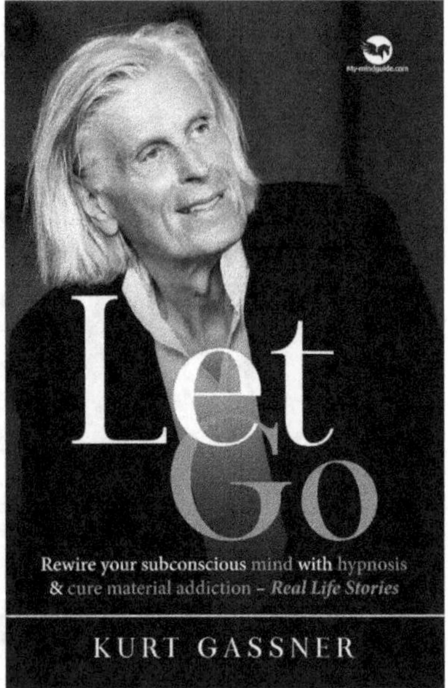

Let
Go
Rewire your subconscious mind with hypnosis
& cure material addiction – Real Life Stories
KURT GASSNER

OTHER BOOKS BY THE AUTHOR

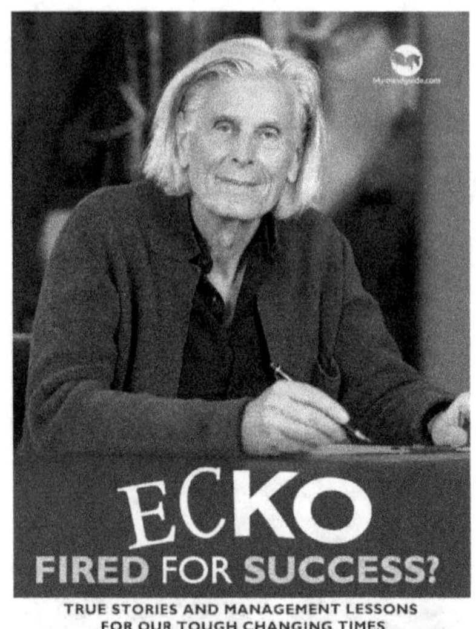

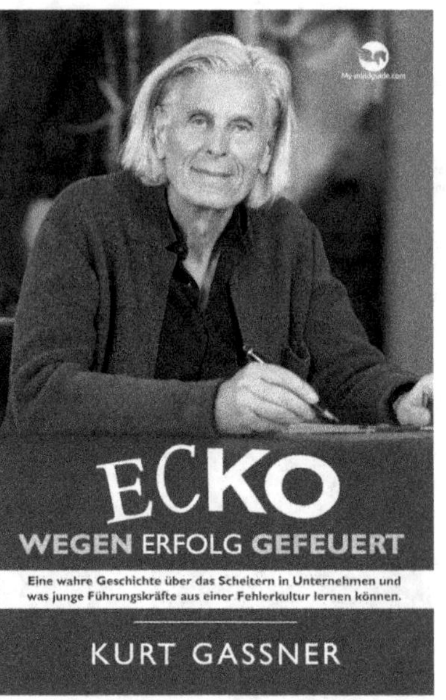

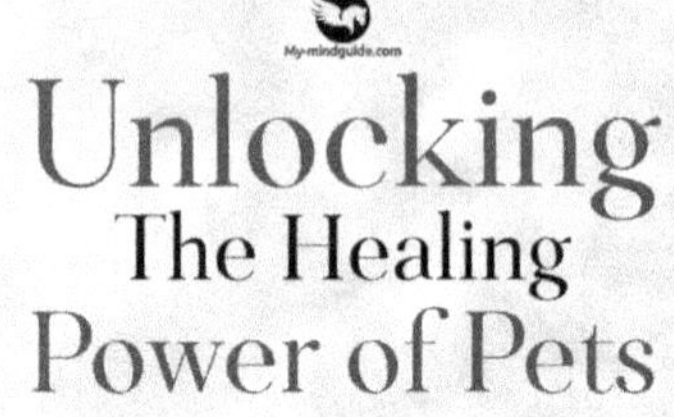

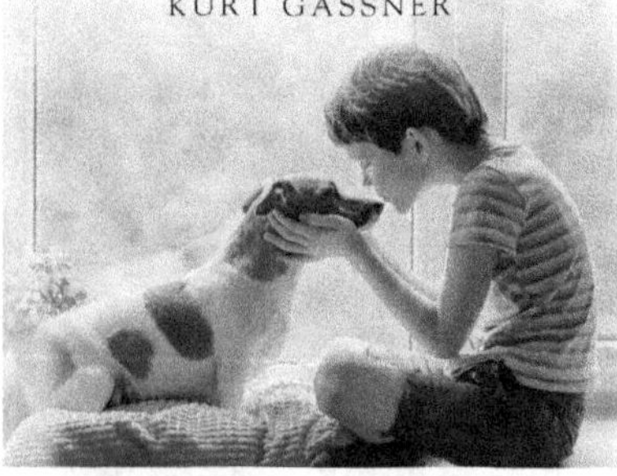

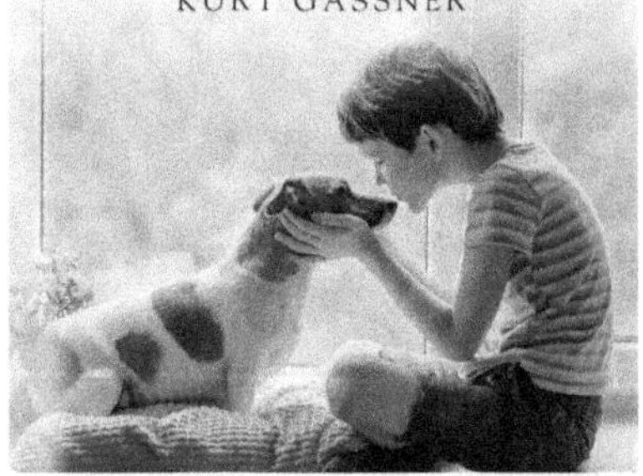

OTHER BOOKS BY THE AUTHOR

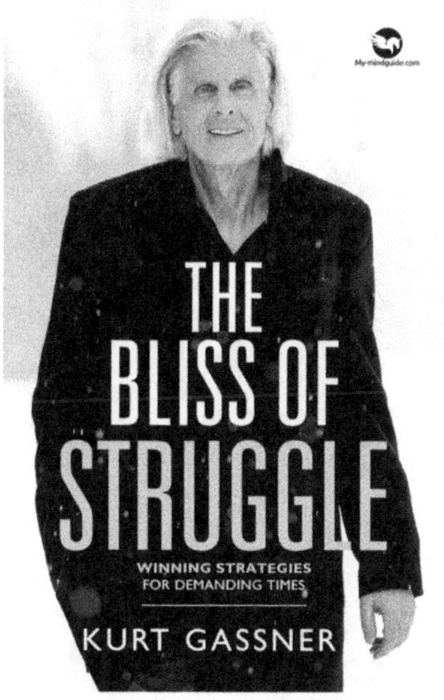

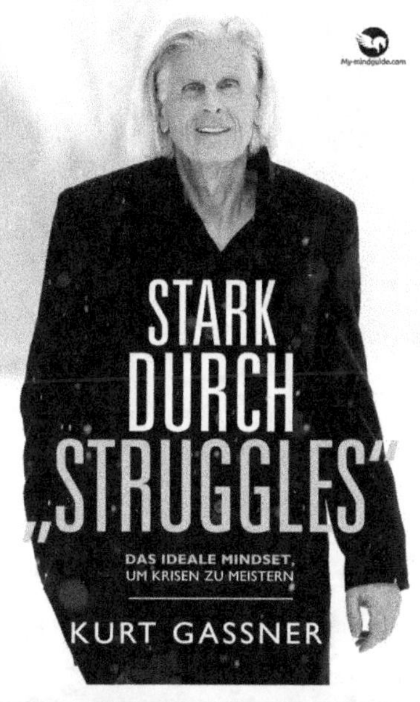

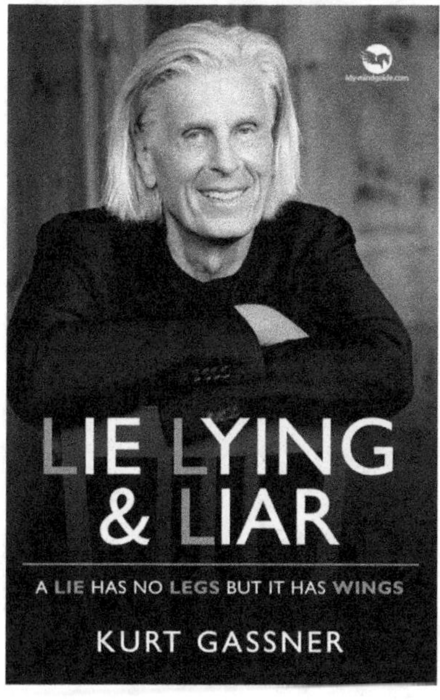

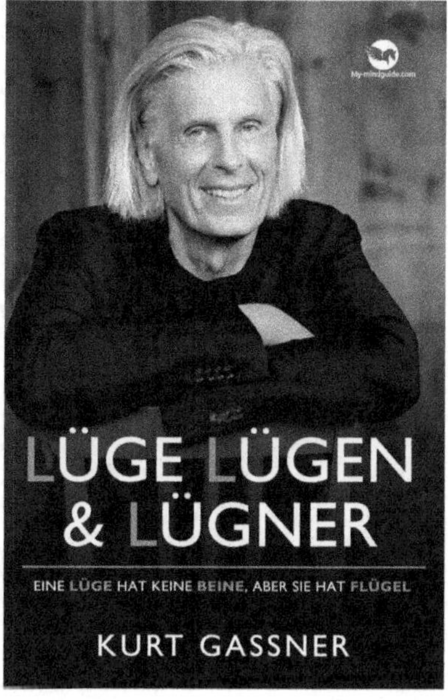

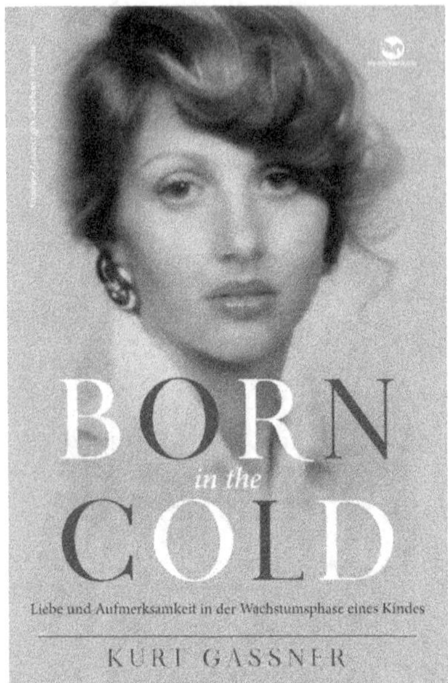

BORN
in the
COLD
Liebe und Aufmerksamkeit in der Wachstumsphase eines Kindes
KURT GASSNER

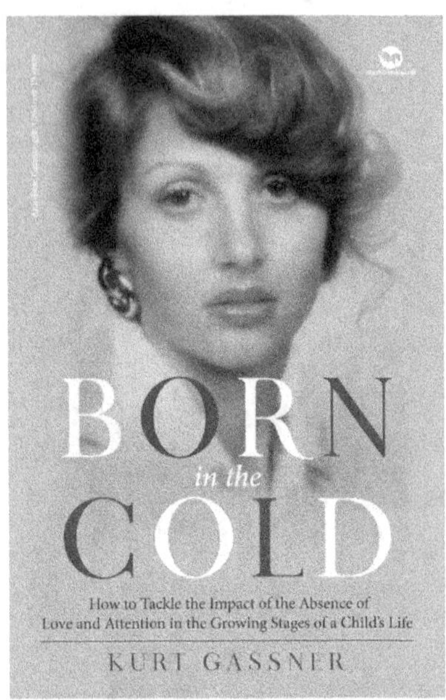

BORN
in the
COLD
How to Tackle the Impact of the Absence of
Love and Attention in the Growing Stages of a Child's Life
KURT GASSNER

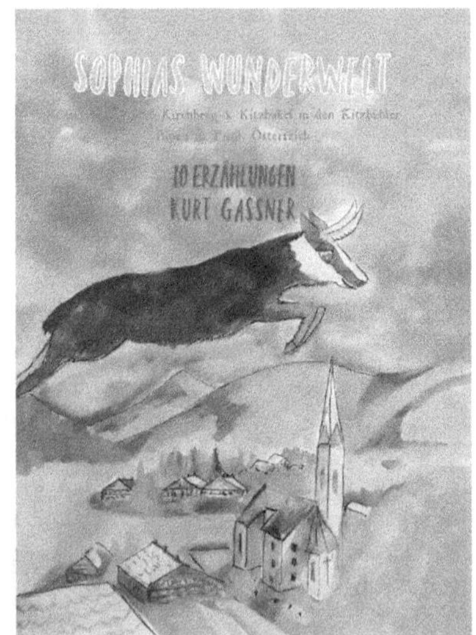

SOPHIAS WUNDERWELT
Kirchberg & Kitzbühel in den Kitzbühler
Alpen in Tirol, Österreich
10 ERZÄHLUNGEN
KURT GASSNER

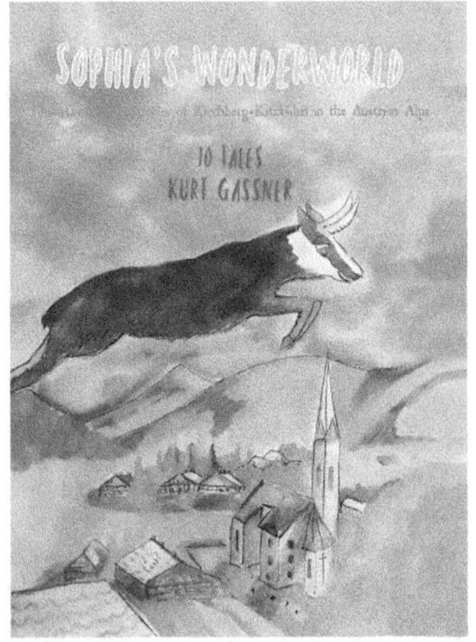

SOPHIA'S WONDERWORLD
of Kirchberg-Kitzbühel in the Austrian Alps
10 TALES
KURT GASSNER

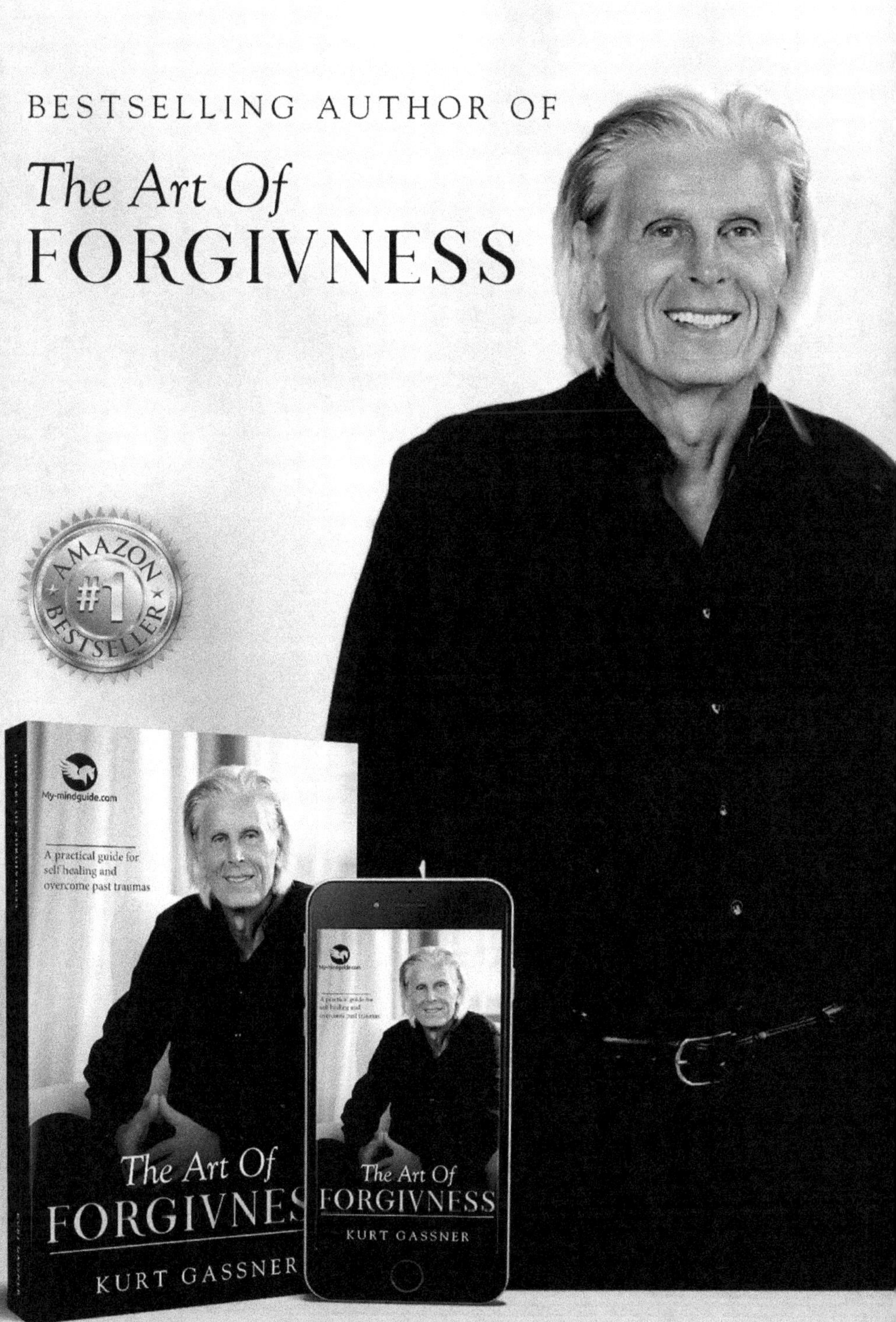

BESTSELLING AUTHOR OF
The Art Of
FORGIVNESS
AMAZON
#1
BESTSELLER
My-mindguide.com
A practical guide for
self healing and
overcome past traumas
The Art Of
FORGIVNESS
KURT GASSNER
The Art Of
FORGIVNESS
KURT GASSNER